International Ophthalmology Clinics

International Ophthalmology Clinics (ISSN 0020-8167) (ISBN 0-316-29399-7). Published quarterly by Little, Brown and Company, 34 Beacon Street, Boston, Massachusetts 02108-1493. Send address changes and subscription orders to Little, Brown and Company, Subscription Department, 34 Beacon St, Boston, MA 02108. Subscription rates per year: personal subscription, U.S. and possessions, $90; foreign (includes Mexico), $116; Canada, $103, PLEASE ADD 7% CANADIAN GST FOR ALL CANADIAN SUBSCRIPTIONS (Registration No. R128537917); institutional, U.S., $113; foreign, $147; Canada, $125. Special rates for students, interns and residents per year: U.S., $61; foreign, $84; Canada, $72. Single copies: $31 for subscribers, $39 for nonsubscribers. In Japan please contact our exclusive agent: Medsi, 1-2-13 Yushima, Bunkyo-ku, Tokyo 113, Japan. Subscription rates per year in Japan: individual, ¥24,200; institutional, ¥28,800 (air cargo service only). Second-class postage paid at Boston, Massachusetts, and at additional mailing offices.

Postmaster: Send address changes to International Ophthalmology Clinics, 34 Beacon St, Boston, MA 02108.

International Ophthalmology Clinics is indexed in Index Medicus, Current Contents/Clinical Practice, Excerpta Medica, and Current Awareness in Biological Sciences.

International Ophthalmology Clinics

Volume 33
Number 1
Winter 1993

New and Evolving Ocular Infections

Little, Brown and Company
BOSTON

Editors

Gilbert Smolin, M.D.
F.I. Proctor Foundation, San Francisco
Department of Ophthalmology,
University of California, San Francisco
Medical Center

Mitchell H. Friedlaender, M.D.
Division of Ophthalmology,
Scripps Clinic and Research Foundation,
La Jolla, California

Editorial Office
1001 Sneath Lane, Room 206
San Bruno, CA 94066

Publisher
Little, Brown and Company, Boston, Massachusetts

Publishing Staff

Editor in Chief
Nancy E. Chorpenning

Executive Editor
David Dionne

Managing Editor
Sherri Frank

Sales and Marketing Manager
Anne Orens

Production Manager
Fredda Purgalin

Contents

Contributing Authors

Sally S. Atherton, Ph.D.
Bascom Palmer Eye Institute
900 N.W. 17th Street
Miami, FL 33101

Cecelia A. Crouse, Ph.D.
Departments of Ophthalmology and Microbiology/
    Immunology
University of Miami
School of Medicine
Miami, FL 33101

William W. Culbertson, M.D.
Bascom Palmer Eye Institute
900 N.W. 17th Street
Miami, FL 33101

Pravin U. Dugel, M.D.
Doheny Eye Institute
1355 San Pablo Street
Los Angeles, CA 90033-1088

Y. Jerold Gordon, M.D.
The Eye and Ear Institute of Pittsburgh
203 Lothrop Street
Pittsburgh, PA 15213

Robert A. Hyndiuk, M.D.
The Eye Institute
8700 W. Wisconsin Avenue
Milwaukee, WI 53226

Dan B. Jones, M.D.
Department of Ophthalmology
Cullen Eye Institute
Baylor College of Medicine
6501 Fannin, NC 200
Houston, TX 77030

Thomas J. Liesegang, M.D.
Department of Ophthalmology
Mayo Clinic Jacksonville
4500 San Pablo Road
Jacksonville, FL 32224

Careen Yen Lowder, M.D., Ph.D.
Department of Ophthalmology
Cleveland Clinic Foundation
9500 Euclid Avenue, A-31
Cleveland, OH 44195

Sid Mandelbaum, M.D.
Department of Clinical Ophthalmology
Long Island Jewish Medical Center
Albert Einstein College of Medicine, *and*
Manhattan Eye, Ear and Throat Hospital
New York, NY
Address correspondence to:
750 Park Avenue
New York, NY 10021

David M. Meisler, M.D.
Department of Ophthalmology
Cleveland Clinic Foundation
9500 Euclid Avenue
Cleveland, OH 44195

Jerry A. Menikoff, M.D.
Department of Ophthalmology
The New York Eye and Ear Infirmary
310 E. 14th Street
New York, NY 10003

Millicent L. Palmer, M.D.
Department of Ophthalmology
University of Arizona
1501 N. Campbell Avenue
Tucson, AZ 85724

Stephen C. Pflugfelder, M.D.
Bascom Palmer Eye Institute
P.O. Box 016880
Miami, FL 33101

Narsing A. Rao, M.D.
Doheny Eye Institute
1355 San Pablo Street
Los Angeles, CA 90033-1088

Olivia N. Serdarevic, M.D.
Department of Ophthalmology
The New York Hospital—CUMC, MEETH
New York, NY, *and*
Hotel-Dieu, University of Paris
Paris, France
Address correspondence to:
103 East 84th Street
New York, NY 10028

Mark G. Speaker, M.D., Ph.D.
Cornea Service
The New York Eye and Ear Infirmary
310 E. 14th Street, Room 401S
New York, NY 10003

George A. Stern, M.D.
Department of Ophthalmology
University of Florida
College of Medicine
Box 100284 JHMHC
Gainesville, FL 32610-0284

Gerald W. Zaidman, M.D.
Department of Ophthalmology
Westchester County Medical Center
Valhalla, NY 10595

Preface

Ocular infections represent an important and challenging aspect of practice for all ophthalmologists. Our ability to recognize and treat ocular infections is constantly being tested as familiar microorganisms undergo changes that allow them to evade the body's immune system and survive within the ocular tissues. Newly recognized infections in individuals immunosuppressed by drugs or disease also present challenges that are being met by new pharmacological agents and innovative methods of drug delivery. This issue of *International Ophthalmology Clinics* focuses on our current understanding of new and evolving ocular infections, as well as recent developments in their diagnosis and treatment.

Mitchell H. Friedlaender

Infectious Crystalline Keratopathy

George A. Stern, M.D.

Infectious crystalline keratopathy (ICK) is an indolent corneal infection in which needlelike, branching, crystalline opacities are seen within the corneal stroma in the absence of appreciable corneal or anterior segment inflammation. The term *crystalline* refers to the appearance of the lesions and does not imply the actual deposition of crystals such as those seen in infantile cystinosis. The majority of these infections occur in corneal grafts, and most are caused by streptococci, particularly the alpha-hemolytic, or viridans, species. In this chapter, I will review the history, diagnosis, microbiological and pathological features, pathogenesis, and treatment of ICK.

■ Historical Background

In 1981, I performed a penetrating keratoplasty on the right eye of a 69-year-old woman with aphakic bullous keratopathy. An 8.0-mm donor button was sutured into a 7.5-mm recipient bed using a continuous 10-0 nylon suture. The donor cornea had been preserved in McCarey-Kaufman medium with gentamicin added. Cultures of the donor rim were negative. The graft rapidly cleared, and the patient was treated with tapering dosages of topical antibiotics and corticosteroids. Five months postoperatively, topical antibiotics were discontinued, and the patient used only dexamethasone sodium phosphate 0.1% once daily. One month later, I began to observe gray-white, branching, needlelike opacities within the peripheral midstroma of the graft, but the transplant was otherwise clear and there were no signs of corneal or anterior segment inflammation. These opacities gradually progressed, and 10 months after operation the patient's visual acuity fell below 20/200 because of extension of the opacities across the visual axis (Fig 1). There were still no signs of corneal or anterior segment inflammation. Eleven months postoperatively, the transplantation was repeated, and the second corneal graft was successful, with no evidence of recurrent infection or inflammation.

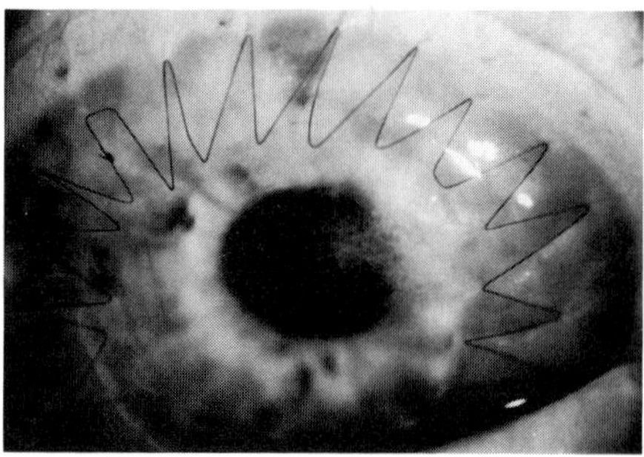

Figure 1 *Infectious crystalline keratopathy from my original case. Gray-white, branching, needlelike crystalline opacities are seen extending across the pupil.*

Histopathological analysis of the donor button, stained with hematoxylin and eosin, revealed a focal area of epithelial ingrowth into the stroma at the site of a suture track. Extending into the stroma from this area of epithelial ingrowth was an intralamellar collection of amorphous basophilic material that, when stained with the Brown and Brenn stain, proved to be colonies of gram-positive cocci (Fig 2). Only rare inflammatory cells were seen. Analysis by transmission electron microscopy confirmed the presence of bacteria. Because infection was not suspected before the histopathological analysis, no cultures of the resected tissue were done.

My colleagues and I [1] reported this case as intrastromal noninflammatory bacterial colonization of a corneal graft, a description that reflected the location of the bacteria and the lack of inflammatory response. We preferred to characterize the process as bacterial colonization rather than infection, believing that the term *infection* should be semantically reserved for inflammation induced by bacteria, whereas *colonization* was the proper term to describe the presence of commensal organisms on or within tissue without inflammation. We speculated that organisms entered the cornea through the suture track, that they were slow-growing and weakly virulent, and that an inflammatory response to the bacteria was suppressed by the long-term use of topical corticosteroids.

In a subsequent report, Meisler and co-workers [2] described 3 similar

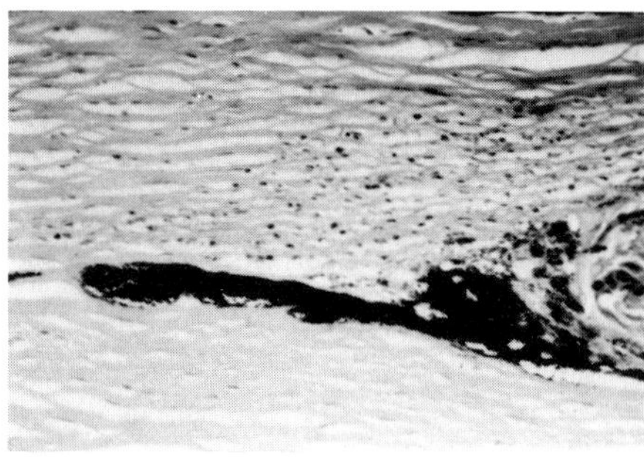

Figure 2 *Photomicrograph of histological section of corneal button from patient shown in Figure 1 (Brown and Brenn stain, original magnification ×40). A large colony of gram-positive cocci is seen extending between stromal lamellae. There is a paucity of inflammatory cells.*

cases and called the entity *infectious crystalline keratopathy*, a term that has persisted to the present time. In addition, these practitioners identified the cause of the infection in 2 of their cases to be alpha-hemolytic streptococci. Since then, there have been numerous studies reported in the ophthalmological literature describing the microbiological features, differential diagnosis, predisposing conditions, pathogenesis, and treatment of ICK.

■ Diagnosis

ICK is characterized by the presence of insidiously progressive graywhite branching opacities within the corneal stroma. These may vary in appearance from small, round stellate opacities to lesions in which large, branching needlelike opacities extend across most of the cornea (Figs 1, 3, 4). The opacities may occur at any depth within the corneal stroma but tend to be isolated within a single lamellar plane. The overlying epithelium is often intact and, despite the infectious nature of the lesions, the eyes exhibit, at most, minimal signs of anterior segment inflammation.

ICK never occurs as a primary disease in a previously healthy cornea. In the vast majority of cases, it occurs as a complication of penetrating keratoplasty or other corneal surgery such as epikeratoplasty [3] or corneal relaxing incisions [4]. Other settings in which ICK has occurred include eyes with postherpetic persistent epithelial defects treated with bandage soft contact lenses [2, 5], *Acanthamoeba* keratitis [6], and topical anesthetic abuse [7]. The lesions often originate at the site of a suture track or at a location from which a loose suture has recently been removed. Nearly all eyes with ICK have been treated with long-term topical corticosteroids and many with topical antimicrobials.

When ICK is suspected, an etiological diagnosis can be made only by culturing infected tissue. In cases where the lesions are very superficial, the causative organisms may be isolated from cultures of routine corneal scrapings. However, because of the depth of the lesions, routine culturing methods often are unsuccessful and corneal biopsies are necessary to con-

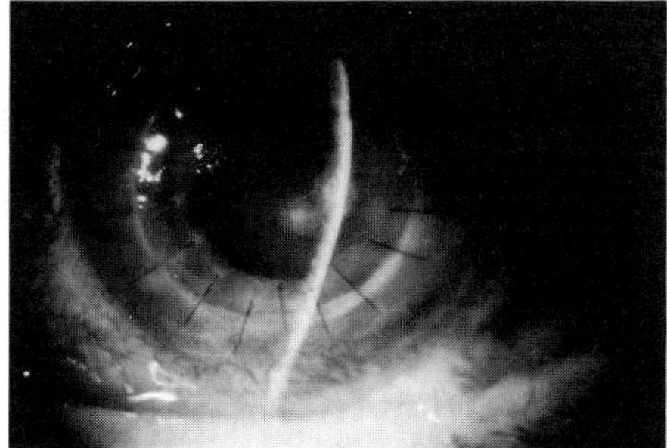

Figure 3 *Infectious crystalline keratopathy in a corneal graft caused by an alphahemolytic streptococcus. In this patient, 2 small round stellate lesions are present in the anterior corneal stroma.*

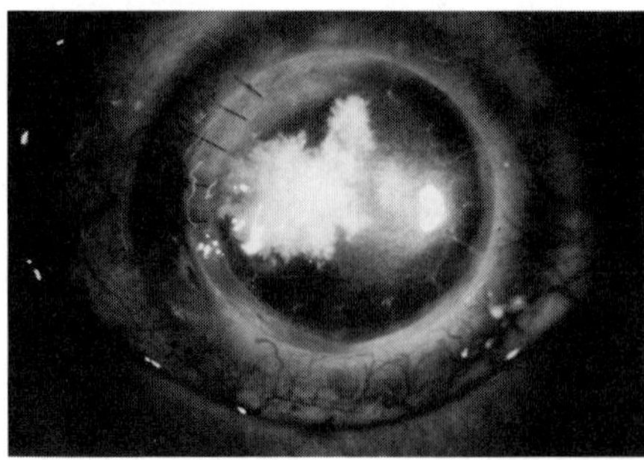

Figure 4 *Infectious crystalline keratopathy in a corneal graft caused by* Candida albicans. *The whitish anterior stromal lesions have a fernlike appearance.*

firm the diagnosis. In many cases, the identification of offending organisms has been made from cultures and histopathological analysis of corneal buttons obtained at the time of repeat corneal transplantations. ICK can be caused by either bacterial or fungal organisms. In addition, this entity has been mimicked by the deposition of calcium into the corneal stroma [8].

■ Microbiological Features

When causative organisms have been isolated, an alpha-hemolytic streptococcus has been the cause of the infection in the majority of cases. Other causative bacteria have included *Peptostreptococcus* [9], nutritionally variant streptococci [10, 11], *Hemophilus aphrophilus* [12], coagulase-negative staphylococci [13, 14], *Pseudomonas maltophilia* [14], *Pseudomonas stutzeri* [14], *Propionibacterium acnes* [14], and mixed infection with *Mycobacterium fortuitum* and *Pseudomonas aeruginosa* [15]. In addition, I have treated an unreported case of ICK caused by *Streptococcus pneumoniae*. Fungi have also been implicated as causes of ICK. These include *Candida albicans* (mixed with *Staphylococcus epidermidis*) [16], *Candida tropicalis* [8], and an unidentified filamentous fungus [8].

■ Treatment

The initial treatment of ICK should consist of intensive topical application of fortified antibiotics that are effective against the causative organisms. Logical choices for treatment of infection caused by alpha-hemolytic streptococci include aqueous penicillin G 100,000 units/ml, cefazolin sodium 50 mg/ml, or vancomycin 10 to 20 mg/ml. Other antibiotics should be considered when different organisms are identified as the cause of the infection. Topical corticosteroids should probably be discontinued. In some cases, the discontinuance of corticosteroids has allowed the crystalline pattern of infection to evolve into a more suppurative process with a better response to treatment [4].

Medical treatment has, however, been generally disappointing. Most cases cured by medical treatment have required prolonged use of antibiotics, and visual results have been poor. In some cases, the prolonged use of topical antibiotics may have caused the emergence of resistant strains of organisms. In addition, the apparently slow replication rate of the organisms may impair the effectiveness of antibiotics that block cell wall synthesis. Envelopment of the organisms in bacterial biofilm [10] or fibrin [17] may limit the bioavailability of antibiotics. More than 50% of cases have failed to respond to medical treatment and have required therapeutic penetrating keratoplasty. Because these eyes have minimal inflammation, therapeutic keratoplasty is generally successful. One case of superficial ICK has been cured by ablation of the infectious lesions with an excimer laser [18].

■ Pathological Features and Pathogenesis

Histopathological studies of ICK have been remarkably consistent in their findings. Characteristically, one finds intralamellar pockets of bacteria within the corneal stroma, generally within a single lamellar plane. Also, there is a surprising paucity of inflammatory cells of any type. The overlying epithelium is often intact if it has not been altered by an accompanying disease process. Collagen lamellae adjacent to the collections of bacteria appear undisturbed, with no evidence of necrosis or corneal thinning. Electron-microscopical analysis of corneal buttons confirms the findings revealed on light microscopy. In addition, bacteria often are seen in varying stages of viability or degeneration. In one study, amorphous material consistent with bacterial biofilm (glycocalyx) was observed surrounding the bacteria [10].

Though there is a great deal of speculation about the pathogenesis of ICK, little is actually known. It is unclear why there is such a predilection for alpha-hemolytic streptococci to cause this infection. These bacteria are the predominant inhabitants of the oral cavity and upper airway, but they rarely are found as part of the normal flora of the eyelids or conjunctiva. Access to the corneal stroma appears to occur via breaks in the corneal surface or through sutures. In our initial case, it was clear that organisms were associated with an epithelial ingrowth at the site of a suture track. In many other cases as well, infection has occurred in association with sutures or at the site of recent suture removal. The common association of ICK with corneal transplantation is likely related to a number of factors commonly found in eyes undergoing corneal surgery, including deep corneal incisions, sutures, persistent epithelial defects (often treated with bandage soft contact lenses), use of topical antibiotics and, most importantly, chronic use of topical corticosteroids.

Once organisms gain access to the corneal stroma, there is surprisingly little inflammation. It appears that organisms causing ICK are minimally virulent. The lack of necrosis adjacent to intrastromal colonies of bacteria suggests that there is little production of destructive bacterial enzymes; more virulent organisms probably cause a more suppurative infection. Also, the indolent nature of the infection suggests that the growth rate of the organisms is slow. It is unclear whether this is due to intrinsic properties of the organisms or whether the corneal stroma provides a marginal environment for bacterial replication. Glycocalyx production may shield the organisms from immune recognition, lessening the inflammatory response. In addition, the chronic use of topical corticosteroids suppresses the inflammatory response; in several clinical cases, the infection has evolved into a more suppurative picture when steroids were discontinued. These latter observations are confirmed in recently developed experimental models of ICK. A crystalline growth pattern was more likely to occur if the bacteria were grown in a medium to enhance glycocalyx production [19], and the crystalline growth pattern was found to occur in eyes treated with corticosteroids, in contrast to corneal abscess formation in eyes not treated with steroids [17].

The reason for the crystalline growth pattern of the lesions is unproved. However, it is probably related to the criss-crossing lamellar architecture of the corneal stroma and represents the path of least resistance to the expanding bacterial colonies.

The poor response to treatment with antibiotics is likely related to a number of factors. Antibiotics that interfere with cell wall synthesis (e.g., penicillins and cephalosporins) require active bacterial replication for their effect; they are much less effective against slowly replicating organisms. In some cases, there may be discrepancies between in vivo and in vitro sensitivities to antibiotics. The nutritionally variant streptococci are relatively resistant when compared to other streptococci [10]. Lastly, as mentioned earlier, the envelopment of the bacteria with biofilms undoubtedly limits the bioavailability of topically administered antibiotics.

This study was supported in part by an unrestricted departmental grant from Research to Prevent Blindness, Inc., New York, NY.

■ References

1. Gorovoy MS, Stern GA, Hood CI, Allen C. Intrastromal noninflammatory bacterial colonization of a corneal graft. Arch Ophthalmol 1983;101:1749–1752
2. Meisler DM, Langston RHS, Naab TJ, et al. Infectious crystalline keratopathy. Am J Ophthalmol 1984;97:337–343

3. Brooks SB, Bruce-Lyle L, Rao NA, Wright KW. Crystalline keratopathy and epikeratophakia. Am J Ophthalmol 1992;113:337–339

4. Kincaid MC, Fouraker BD, Schanzlin DJ. Infectious crystalline keratopathy after relaxing incisions. Am J Ophthalmol 1991;111:374–375

5. Zabel RW, Mintsioulis G, MacDonald I, Tuft S. Infectious crystalline keratopathy. Can J Ophthalmol 1988;23:311–314

6. Davis RM, Schroeder RP, Rowsey JJ, et al. *Acanthamoeba* keratitis and infectious crystalline keratopathy. Arch Ophthalmol 1987;105:1524–1527

7. Kintner JC, Grossniklaus HE, Lass JH, Jacobs G. Infectious crystalline keratopathy associated with topical anesthetic abuse. Cornea 1990;9:77–80

8. Weisenthal RW, Krachmer JH, Folberg R, et al. Postkeratoplasty crystalline deposits mimicking bacterial infectious crystalline keratopathy. Am J Ophthalmol 1988;105:70–74

9. Eiferman RA, Ogden LL, Snyder J. Anaerobic peptostreptococcal keratitis. Am J Ophthalmol 1985;100:335–336

10. Ormerod LD, Ruoff KL, Meisler DM, et al. Infectious crystalline keratopathy. Role of nutritionally variant streptococci and other bacterial factors. Ophthalmology 1991;98:159–169

11. Townshend L, Slomovic A, Hunter W. Infectious crystalline keratopathy. Can J Ophthalmol 1989;24:325–326

12. Groden LR, Pascucci SE, Brinser JH. *Hemophilus aphrophilus* as a cause of crystalline keratopathy. Am J Ophthalmol 1987;104:89–90

13. Lubniewski AJ, Houchin KW, Holland EJ, et al. Posterior infectious crystalline keratopathy with *Staphylococcus epidermidis*. Ophthalmology 1990;97:1454–1459

14. Rabinowitz SM, Alfonso E, Culbertson WW, et al. Infectious crystalline keratopathy—a report of ten cases and presentation of new clinical observations. Invest Ophthalmol Vis Sci 1989;30(suppl):276

15. Hu FR. Infectious crystalline keratopathy caused by *Mycobacterium fortuitum* and *Pseudomonas aeruginosa*. Am J Ophthalmol 1990;109:738–739

16. Wilhelmus KR, Robinson NM. Infectious crystalline keratopathy caused by *Candida albicans*. Am J Ophthalmol 1991;112:322–325

17. McDonnell PJ, Kwitko S, McDonnell JM, et al. Characterization of infectious crystalline keratitis caused by a human isolate of *Streptococcus mitis*. Arch Ophthalmol 1991;109:1147–1151

18. Eiferman RA, Forgey DR, Cook YD. Excimer laser ablation of infectious crystalline keratopathy. Arch Ophthalmol 1992;110:18

19. Hunts J, Matoba A, Osato M. Induction of infectious crystalline keratopathy is influenced by growth conditions of the infecting organism. Invest Ophthalmol Vis Sci 1992;33(suppl):937

The Ocular Manifestations of Lyme Disease

Gerald W. Zaidman, M.D.

Lyme disease is the most common arthropod-related disease in the United States and Europe [1]. Its name derives from the city of Lyme, Connecticut, where in 1975, a group of mothers observed a geographical clustering of juvenile arthritis in their community and alerted local health authorities. Dr. Allen Steere and his colleagues at the Yale University School of Medicine then described a syndrome of acute arthritis usually preceded by an expanding red rash (erythema chronicum migrans [ECM]) after an insect bite. They found that the disease occurred predominantly in the summer and early fall.

Recognition that the ECM rash, originally described in 1909 in Sweden in patients bitten by ticks of the *Ixodes* genus, was part of Lyme disease led to the realization that *Ixodes* ticks were involved in spreading the disease. In 1982, Drs. Burgdorfer and Barbour isolated a new spirochete, called *Borrelia burgdorferi*, from the *I. dammini* tick. Later, the same spirochete was cultured from the skin, blood, and cerebrospinal fluid of patients infected with Lyme disease [2]. Thus, Lyme disease, or Lyme borreliosis, came to be recognized as a systemic spirochetal infection with many clinical manifestations. It is now considered similar to another spirochetal infection, syphilis, in its multisystemic involvement, multiple stages, and ability to mimic other diseases.

■ Epidemiological Features

Since it was originally described, Lyme disease has steadily increased in incidence. Over the last 10 years, the number of reported cases has increased from fewer than 500 in 1982 to more than 7,500 in 1989 [3]. It has now been reported in 43 of the 50 states in the United States. Lyme disease clusters in three geographical areas in the United States: the Northeast, especially in southern Connecticut, Westchester County of New York State, and Long Island; the Midwest, mainly Wisconsin and Minnesota;

and the Northwest, mainly Washington, Oregon, and northern California. These areas correspond to the distribution of the *Ixodes* ticks; the *I. dammini* in the East and Midwest and the *I. pacificus* in the Northwest. In Europe, it is carried by the *I. ricinus* tick, and the disease is most frequently seen in Germany, Austria, Switzerland, France, and Sweden. Recently, the disease has also been reported in Asia (especially Hokkaido, Japan, in association with *I. persulcatus* and *I. ovatus*) [4] and in Australia.

The disease is transmitted to humans by the bite of an infected tick. The tick life cycle consists of three stages (Fig 1). The first two, larval and nymphal, are immature stages. In these, the tick's preferred host in the United States is the white-footed mouse (*Peromyscus leucopus*). These mice apparently are immune to the spirochetal infection. In its adult form (the third stage), the preferred host is the white-tailed deer. However, at any stage of its life cycle, the tick can take its blood meal by biting humans or other mammals.

The nymphal stage of the tick is the most aggressive. This stage gener-

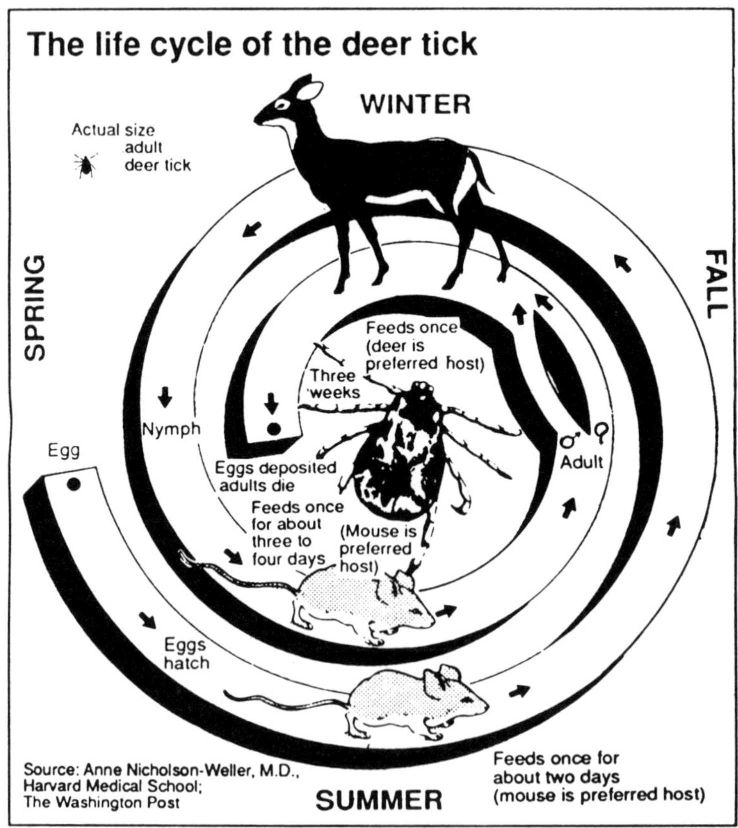

Figure 1 *The life cycle of a deer tick.*

ally feeds in May, June, or July. It is because of the extremely small size of the nymphal stage of the tick (smaller than a pencil point) that many people do not remember the tick bite. The adult tick, which is larger and more recognizable, generally feeds on larger animals or people in the early fall.

■ Clinical Manifestations

The clinical manifestations of classical, untreated, Lyme disease occurs in three stages [1]. Stage 1 is the localized bull's-eye skin rash of ECM. Stage 2 follows weeks or months later with varied systemic symptoms. Stage 3 consists of late chronic arthritis. However, the symptoms in each stage can overlap, and many patients do not recall or manifest each stage [5]. Therefore, a preferable classification, analogous to that used in classifying syphilis, divides Lyme disease into early and late infectious stages (Table 1). The early infection comprises stages 1 and 2 and includes that period of intermittent symptoms weeks or months after the onset of the disease. Late infection, or stage 3, begins many months to a year after onset.

Localized Early Infection (Stage 1)

Stage 1 manifests soon after the tick bite and consists of the pathognomonic skin rash, ECM (Fig 2). This rash is the hallmark of the disease and begins 3 to 30 days after the tick bite. However, only 60 to 80% of patients have the rash, and fewer than half of the patients recall the bite [2].

The rash usually occurs in the thigh, groin, or axilla. It begins as a red macule or papule that quickly, over a few days, expands in a circular fashion. Frequently, there is an area of central clearing, thus giving the

Table 1   *Classification of Lyme Disease and its Manifestations*

Early infection
Localized (stage 1)
  Erythema chronicum migrans (ECM)
  Flulike symptoms
Disseminated (stage 2)
  Relapsing migratory arthritis or monoarthritis
  Neurological disease (cranial neuropathy, meningitis, radiculopathy)
  Cardiac atrioventricular block
  Ocular manifestations
Late infection
Persistent (stage 3)
  Prolonged chronic arthritis
  Chronic neurological syndromes
  Ocular manifestations

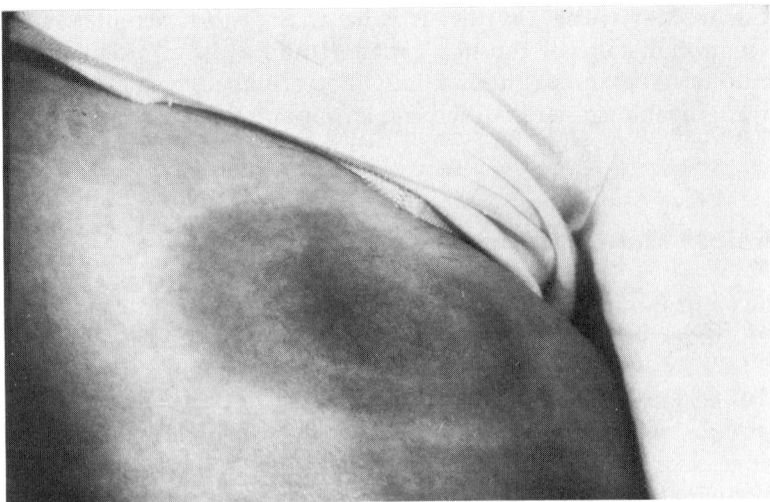

Figure 2 *Erythema chronicum migrans.*

classical bull's-eye appearance. The rash can vary in size from 2 to 60 cm. It is commonly accompanied by flulike constitutional symptoms consisting of headache, fever, chills, myalgias, or arthralgias. Though some patients can have severe symptoms, most, even if not treated, have a mild disease with fading of the rash within 1 month.

Disseminated Early Infection (Stage 2)

In some untreated patients, a presumed spirochetemia occurs days or weeks after inoculation [6]. Some of these patients will develop signs and symptoms of serious organ involvement. Among such patients, the major problems seen are neurological (in 15% of patients) cardiac (in 8% of patients), and arthritic (in 60% of patients). Neurological disease includes cranial neuropathy (especially Bell's palsy), aseptic meningitis, headache, encephalitis, or peripheral neuritis. These symptoms are often transient and mild.

Cardiac disease is usually brief and mild, typically consisting of fluctuating degrees of atrioventricular block. Rarely, some patients develop severe myopericarditis. The most important problem is the arthritis, which usually is acute and severe. Typically, it involves one or a few joints, usually the knees, shoulders, or ankles. It is characterized by recurrences and relapses.

Symptoms in these patients occur several weeks to months after inoculation. It is during this stage that severe ophthalmic manifestations (diplopia, cranial nerve palsies, optic neuritis, etc.) first occur.

Persistent Late Infection (Stage 3)

Although there is a great deal of variability, a small group of patients have intermittent symptoms beyond the second stage. They may develop persistent disease. The most common late disorder is chronic Lyme arthritis, a severe relapsing chronic arthritis that, in some patients, may lead to permanent joint disability. Some patients may also have one of several types of chronic neurological syndromes of the central or peripheral nervous system. These include neuropsychiatric disease, radiculopathy, chronic fatigue, peripheral neuropathy, or memory loss. Acrodermatitis chronica atrophicans may also occur. The only ocular manifestations that have been described in this stage are keratitis and posterior segment inflammatory disease.

■ Ocular Manifestations

Ocular manifestations of Lyme disease have involved every portion of the eye. A review of the literature indicates that, as in many other spirochetal infections, the ocular manifestations of Lyme disease vary depending on the stage of the disease (Table 2).

In stage 1 Lyme disease, the only ocular manifestations are conjunctivitis and photophobia. Overall, these are the most common manifestations, occurring in up to 11% of patients [1]. The conjunctivitis has not been well described, but it appears to be a nonspecific conjunctival inflammation that resolves without treatment. Because of its mild and brief nature, ophthalmologists are usually not consulted.

It is during stage 2 (disseminated infection) of Lyme disease that significant ophthalmic complications first appear. Therefore, it is during this stage that an ophthalmologist is most likely to see a patient with Lyme disease.

The most common ophthalmic presentations of stage 2 Lyme disease are various neuroophthalmological manifestations. Typically, these are seventh cranial nerve palsy (Bell's palsy), other cranial nerve palsies causing diplopia, blurred vision, and headache. Most of these patients will exhibit a concurrent neurological complication of Lyme disease as well, usually aseptic meningitis or radiculopathy. Ophthalmologists may find that some patients with stage 2 disease will present with the typical triad of Lyme neuroborreliosis, consisting of cranial nerve palsies, meningitis, and radiculopathy.

Clark and colleagues [7], in a series of 951 patients with Lyme disease, found that 10.6% had seventh nerve paresis or Bell's palsy. Most of these patients had unilateral disease, but nearly one-fourth had bilateral Bell's palsy. In general, symptoms occurred within 1 month of the skin rash and usually during the summer. Eighty-five percent of the patients recalled the

Table 2 *Ocular Manifestations of Lyme Disease*

Early infection
Localized (stage 1)
  Conjunctivitis
  Photophobia
Disseminated (stage 2)
  Neuroophthalmological disorders
    Bell's palsy
    Cranial neuropathy and diplopia
    Disc edema and blurred vision
    Headache
  Posterior segment inflammatory disease (see under "Late Infection")
Late infection
Persistent (stage 3)
  Anterior segment inflammatory disease
    Episcleritis
    Symblepharon
    Keratitis
  Posterior segment inflammatory disease (which may occur also in stage 2)
    Iritis
    Pars planitis
    Vitritis
    Choroiditis
    Panuveitis
    Retinal vasculitis
    Exudative retinal detachment
    Branch retinal artery occlusion

skin rash, whereas only 38% remembered the tick bite. One-third of the patients had various neurological symptoms. Appropriate treatment avoided the complications of exposure keratitis or corneal abrasions. In 99% of the patients, the paralysis totally resolved without sequelae. The median time to recovery was 1 month.

Diplopia is typically due to sixth nerve paresis. However, third and fourth cranial nerve deficits have been seen [8]. These palsies can occur individually or in combination, and they are usually associated with other neurological abnormalities. Most appear to resolve without sequelae within 2 weeks to 5 months after onset.

Blurred vision can also be seen during this stage. Complaints of blurred vision should lead to a search for papilledema, optic or retrobulbar neuritis, and pseudotumor cerebri. The optic nerve disease may be unilateral or bilateral. These may be solitary findings, but they can also be seen in association with aseptic meningitis, headache, and cranial nerve abnormalities [8, 9]. Patients may also complain of decreased color vision and visual field changes. Also, because some of the cases of papilledema are associated with increased intracranial pressure [10], a complete neuroophthalmological workup, including cranial tomography, is indicated in patients with Lyme papilledema.

There are anecdotal reports that some patients with optic nerve disease may progress to optic atrophy and loss of vision or of their visual field. In these few cases, it appears that appropriate therapy prevents permanent visual sequelae. There have also been case reports of patients with reversible Horner's syndrome [11], orbital myositis [12], and temporal arteritis [13] in association with Lyme disease.

It is in late stage 2 or in stage 3 (persistent infection) that most of the severe ocular manifestations of Lyme disease are seen. These include episcleritis [14], symblepharon [15], keratitis [16, 17], iritis, pars planitis [18], vitritis, choroiditis [19], panuveitis [20], retinal vasculitis [21], exudative retinal detachment [19], and branch retinal artery occlusion [22]. Of this group of inflammatory disorders, keratitis and vitritis and pars planitis appear to be the most common.

The keratitis associated with Lyme disease is seen only during stage 3 and generally presents several years after inoculation. Typically, the patient complains of mild blurring of vision and occasional photophobia [16, 17, 23]. On examination (Fig 3), one typically sees a bilateral patchy, stromal keratitis. The entire stroma may be involved, with scattered focal nummular opacities. Other presentations reported include peripheral keratitis and peripheral stromal edema with mild corneal neovascularization [17, 24]. The keratitis is similar to, though milder than, that reported in syphilitic keratitis [16].

Posterior segment inflammatory disease is difficult to categorize because it can present either in late stage 2 or in stage 3 disease. It generally presents as a bilateral pars planitis associated with granulomatous iridocyclitis and vitritis [18]. Most of the patients have a history of prior systemic or ocular manifestations of Lyme disease. The pars planitis is atypical in that most patients also have granulomatous keratic precipitates and poste-

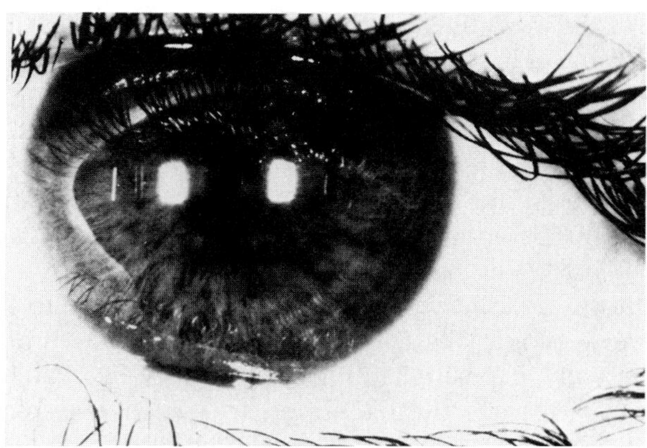

Figure 3 *Slit-lamp photograph of a patient with Lyme keratitis. Scattered nummular opacities are present.*

rior synechiae. The vitritis usually consists of multiple inflammatory nodules or "snowbank exudates." Some patients can progress to retinal vasculitis, choroiditis, exudative retinal detachment, and vitreous hemorrhage. One patient developed a branch retinal artery occlusion. Another developed progressive panophthalmitis and a phthisical eye [9].

In general, if a patient from an area endemic with Lyme disease presents with a syndrome resembling pars planitis and complicated by posterior synechiae and granulomatous uveitis, Lyme disease should be considered.

Laboratory Tests

Because many patients with suspected Lyme disease do not recall the tick bite or the skin rash, laboratory tests have become very important in establishing the diagnosis. However, there is a great deal of difficulty and confusion in the interpretation of the various tests used for Lyme disease. The ideal and definitive test would be culture and isolation of *B. burgdorferi* from a patient suspected of having Lyme disease, but this is very difficult and expensive. Currently, therefore, serological workup is the most practical diagnostic aid. The two most frequently used serological tests are the immunofluorescent assay (IFA) and the enzyme-linked immunosorbent assay (ELISA). Most laboratories now prefer the ELISA test because it is more specific and sensitive [1, 2]. However, since serological testing is not yet standardized, many laboratories are still only able to perform the IFA [25].

The results obtained on the same patient can vary from laboratory to laboratory. A recent study in New Jersey indicated that there was only a 50% correlation between laboratories on serological testing for Lyme disease [26]. Another study demonstrated that of 17 patients with any positive serological test for Lyme disease, 9 had a positive IFA and ELISA, 5 had a positive IFA and a negative ELISA, and 3 had a positive ELISA and a negative IFA [27]. Such variation among laboratories are due to a lack of standardization; different laboratories use different antigens, prepare similar antigens differently, absorb competing antigens differently, and use different normal values.

Additionally, it is not uncommon to have false-negative or false-positive serologies. False-negative tests are generally seen during the first several weeks of infection [1, 18]. Most patients, during the acute phase (stage 1), have not mustered sufficient antibody response to Lyme disease to give a positive serological test. By 5 weeks after disease onset, however, 90% of patients will be positive for either ELISA or IFA [8, 28]. With longer duration of disease, the likelihood for positive serological testing increases (Table 3).

Another important cause of false-negative tests are patients who have been partially or inadequately treated with oral antibiotics early in Lyme disease [1, 2, 28]. These patients may never develop positive serological tests but may develop chronic symptoms. Also, immunosuppressed patients unable to muster an antibody response can be falsely negative.

False-positive tests are due to serological cross-reactivity. Cross-reactivity has been reported between Lyme disease and syphilis, Rocky Mountain spotted fever, leptospirosis, relapsing fever, some autoimmune diseases, yaws, and pinta [4, 8, 28, 29]. The cross-reaction between Lyme disease and syphilis is clinically the most important and has been reported in anywhere from 22 to 54% of patients [29].

To improve our diagnostic capability, other laboratory tests have been proposed, including immunoblotting (Western blot), T-lymphocyte cell assay, urine antigen assay, biopsy, and polymerase chain reaction (PCR) [8, 25, 28]. Of this group, the only test currently of any clinical significance is the Western blot, which is more specific and sensitive than ELISA. Researchers hope that this test will be improved to provide true positive results in the early phases of the disease, though currently it is usually negative. In contrast to IFA and ELISA, however, it is 100% positive in stages 2 and 3 (see Table 4). Nonetheless, the Western blot is much more difficult to perform than these assays, and only a few laboratories are set up for it.

The only other test occasionally used is the PCR, which is specific for *B. burgdorferi*. However, it is also expensive, easily contaminated (thereby causing a high number of false-positive results), and generally unavailable.

The best current recommendation is that whenever Lyme disease is suspected, one should order four tests—Lyme IFA, Lyme ELISA, the Venereal Disease Research Laboratory test (VDRL), and the fluorescent treponemal antibody absorption test (FTA-ABS) [30]. The results should be interpreted with caution and always in association with the patient's clinical manifestations. In our laboratories, an IFA titer of more than or equal to 1 : 256 and an ELISA titer of more than or equal to 1.2 is considered significant.

■ Diagnosis

General Principles

The systemic and ocular manifestations of Lyme disease may mimic many diseases. Most importantly, it mimics many of the diverse clinical manifestations of syphilis, but viral syndromes, juvenile rheumatoid arthritis, infectious mononucleosis, mumps, multiple sclerosis, amyotrophic lateral sclerosis, or infectious arthritis can all give similar clinical findings. Nonetheless, the diagnosis is not difficult if one maintains a high index of suspicion and follows the recommendations of the Centers for Disease Control (Table 4) [2]. If a patient comes from an area endemic for Lyme disease or has traveled in such an area, one should suspect Lyme disease

Table 3 *Laboratory Tests for Lyme Disease*

Test	Early infection		Late infection
	Stage 1	Stage 2	Stage 3
ELISA	Negative	90% Positive	100% Positive
IFA	Negative	90% Positive	100% Positive
Western blot	Negative	100% Positive	100% Positive

ELISA = enzyme-linked immunosorbent assay; *IFA* = immunofluorescent assay.

in any patient with a history of ECM. If there is no history of a rash, a patient from an endemic area who has ocular or systemic symptoms consistent with Lyme disease (arthritis, Bell's palsy, aseptic meningitis, optic neuritis, pars planitis, keratitis, etc.) and a positive serological workup probably has Lyme disease. Evidence of the disease should also be sought in patients from an endemic area with equivocal serological studies and involvement of two or more organ systems.

In a nonendemic area, to make the diagnosis of Lyme disease the Centers for Disease Control require ECM plus a positive serological profile, or ECM with systemic or ocular manifestations involving two or more organ systems or, in the absence of ECM, a positive serological profile and involvement of two or more organ systems. For the ophthalmologist, any patient who presents with a cranial neuropathy (especially Bell's palsy), unexplained keratitis, idiopathic chronic uveitis, pars planitis, inflammatory optic nerve disease, or unexplained papilledema should be questioned about a history of a tick bite, skin rash, recurrent arthritis, or aseptic meningitis. One should also inquire whether the patient has been in an area endemic for Lyme disease. A positive answer to any of these questions is an indication for serological testing. However, since seronegative Lyme disease does occur, the diagnosis of Lyme disease should depend on clinical considerations and not solely on the serological workup.

Table 4 *Diagnostic Criteria for Lyme Disease*

Endemic area
Erythema chronicum migrans (ECM)
Positive serological profile and involvement of ≥ 1 organ system
Positive or negative serological profile and involvement of ≥ 2 organ systems

Nonendemic area
ECM with positive serological profile
ECM and involvement of ≥ 2 organ systems
Positive serological profile and involvement of ≥ 2 organ systems

Table 5   *Treatment of Lyme Disease*

Early (stage 1, stage 2)
Oral tetracycline (doxycycline), penicillin (amoxicillin), or erythromycin for 3 weeks
  (30 days for stage 2)
Late (severe stage 2, stage 3)
Intravenous penicillin G or ceftriaxone for 14 days

■ Treatment

The pathogenesis of Lyme disease is unclear. Debate continues over whether manifestations of Lyme disease are due to infectious proliferation of the organism (via hematogenous spread) or secondary to immunological phenomena. There is consensus that stage 1 Lyme disease is probably due to infectious spread of the organism. However, the later stages may be immune-mediated, secondary to an active infection, or due to a vasculitis [8]. Therefore, the best therapeutic approach is controversial.

Despite the lack of controlled studies on the optimal treatment of Lyme disease, there is agreement that all patients with stage 1 Lyme disease should be treated with oral antibiotics (Table 5). The role of antibiotics during early infection is to eradicate the organism and to prevent later complications. Research on the in vitro susceptibility of the organism has provided some guidelines to therapy [31]. The indolent nature of the *Borrelia* organism and its similarity to other spirochetes have predisposed physicians to the prolonged use of antibiotics to achieve adequate blood levels [2]. Therefore, once a diagnosis is made (or considered), in adults and nonpregnant women stage 1 Lyme disease is treated with 2 to 3 weeks of oral tetracycline, 500 mg four times daily; doxycycline, 100 mg twice daily; phenoxymethyl penicillin, 500 mg four times daily; or amoxicillin, 500 mg three to four times per day [1, 2, 5, 31]. Patients who cannot tolerate tetracycline (i.e., children, pregnant women) or who are allergic to penicillin are given erythromycin, 500 mg four times per day. The duration of treatment is somewhat empirical, depending on the patient's clinical response, and some physicians advocate longer treatment regimens.

For later stages of Lyme disease, the treatment depends on disease severity. Mild neurological disorders (headache, Bell's palsy) and mild arthralgias can be treated with oral antibiotics, but patients usually need 30 days of therapy. Patients with severe disease (meningitis, carditis, etc.) require parenteral therapy, either 14 days of intravenous penicillin G, 3 to 4 million units every 4 hours, or intravenous ceftriaxone, 2 gm/day in divided doses. Finally, all patients should be observed for a possible Jarisch-Herxheimer reaction shortly after instituting therapy.

Because of the paucity of cases of ocular Lyme disease, the acceptable treatment of the ocular manifestations is unclear. Stage 1 conjunctivitis and photophobia require no therapy. Stage 2 Bell's palsy is self-limiting

[7] and, other than supportive therapy to prevent the complications of Bell's palsy and exposure keratitis, no topical antibiotic therapy is needed. If the patient has never received oral antibiotic therapy for his or her disease, then 30 days of tetracycline or penicillin should be administered to avoid further complications of the disease.

Keratitis and episcleritis have been shown to benefit from topical corticosteroids [14–17]. Since this is probably an autoimmue disorder and is limited to the anterior segment, a short course of prednisolone acetate 1% or fluorometholone 0.1% four times daily is used. Improvement is usually seen within several weeks to months, at which time the topical corticosteroids can be tapered. They can be reinstituted for any recurrence. Systemic antibiotic therapy is indicated if the patient has never received any systemic treatment.

The best treatment regimen for severe neuroophthalmic disease (involving the optic nerve) or posterior segment disease (pars planitis, vitritis, choroiditis, etc.) has not been established. Oral corticosteroids without concomitant antibiotics should not be used in the treatment of these complications. Prior treatment with oral corticosteroids may, in fact, make eradication of the organism more difficult [18]. It appears that the best approach for patients with these severe ocular complications of Lyme disease is the "therapeutic antibiotic trial" [18]. Patients with clinically suspected late-stage severe ocular Lyme disease should be given 2 weeks of intravenous penicillin or ceftriaxone (or 30 days of oral tetracycline). The dose regimen should be the same as for the treatment of patients with the late stages of systemic Lyme disease. Most patients treated in this fashion respond with successful resolution of their ocular disease. If the patient responds to treatment, ocular Lyme disease is diagnosed and no further therapy is needed. A negative therapeutic trial should lead one to search for an alternative diagnosis.

■ Summary

Lyme disease (with its ocular manifestations) is a worldwide disorder that is rapidly increasing in frequency. It is a treatable, multisystemic disease that presents in three stages of severity. It can present with unusual forms of conjunctivitis, keratitis, cranial nerve palsies, optic nerve disease, uveitis, vitritis, and other forms of posterior segment inflammatory disease. A patient with any of these ocular manifestations should be questioned for exposure to an area endemic for Lyme disease, tick bites, skin rash, or arthritis. Such patients should undergo serological testing. If the clinical presentation is suggestive of Lyme disease, a course of oral antibiotics should be used (unless the patient gives a history of adequate therapy). Topical corticosteroids can be used for anterior segment inflammation. An antibiotic therapeutic trial can be used for posterior segment or neuroophthalmic disease. Systemic corticosteroids without concomitant antibiotics should not be used in the treatment of ocular Lyme disease. If ocular Lyme disease is discovered and treated early, response to therapy is usually satisfactory.

■ References

1. Steere AC. Medical progress—Lyme disease. N Engl J Med 1989;321:586–596
2. Weinstein A, Bujak DI. Lyme disease: a review of its clinical features. NY State J Med 1989;89:566–571
3. Altman LK. Genetic factors emerge as key to onset of Lyme arthritis. NY Times, 3 July 1990
4. Isogai E, Isogai H, Kotake S, et al. Detection of antibodies against *Borrelia burgdorferi* in patients with uveitis. Am J Ophthalmol 1991;112:23–30
5. Nadelman RB, Wormser GP. A clinical approach to Lyme disease. Mt. Sinai J Med 1990;57:144–156
6. Luft BJ, Steinman CR, Neimaik HC, et al. Invasion of the central nervous system by *Borrelia burgdorferi* in acute disseminated infection. JAMA 1992;267:1364–1367
7. Clark JR, Carlson RD, Sasaki CT, et al. Facial paralysis in Lyme disease. Laryngoscope 1985;95:1341–1345
8. Lesser RL, Kornmehl EW, Pachmer AR, et al. Neuroophthalmologic manifestations of Lyme disease. Ophthalmology 1990;97:699–706
9. Kauffmann DJH, Wormser GP. Ocular Lyme disease: case report and review of the literature. Br J Ophthalmol 1990;74:325–327
10. Jacobson DM, Freus DB. Pseudotumor cerebri syndrome associated with Lyme disease. Am J Ophthalmol 1989;106:81–82
11. Glauser TA, Brennan PJ, Galetta, SL. Reversible Horner's syndrome and Lyme disease. J Clin Neuro Ophthalmol 1989;9:225–228
12. Seidenberg KB, Leib ML. Orbital myositis with Lyme disease. Am J Ophthalmol 1990;109:13–16
13. Pizzarello LD, MacDonald AB, Seinlear R, et al. Temporal arteritis associated with *Borrelia* infection. A case report. J Clin Neuro Ophthalmol 1989;9:3–6
14. Flack AJ, Lavoie PE. Episcleritis, conjunctivitis and keratitis as ocular manifestations of Lyme disease. Ophthalmology 1990;97:973–975
15. Zaidman GW. Episcleritis and symblepharon associated with Lyme keratitis. Am J Ophthalmol 1990;109:487–488
16. Baum J, Barza M, Weinstein P, et al. Bilateral keratitis as a manifestation of Lyme disease. Am J Ophthalmol 1988;105:75–77
17. Kornmehl EW, Lesser RL, Jaros P, et al. Bilateral keratitis in Lyme disease. Ophthalmology 1989;96:1194–1197
18. Winward KE, Lawton Smith J, Culbertson WW, Paris-Hamelin A. Ocular Lyme borreliosis. Am J Ophthalmol 1989;108:651–657
19. Bialasiewicz AA, Ruprecht KW, Nauman GOH, Blenk H. Bilateral diffuse choroiditis and exudative retinal detachments with evidence of Lyme disease. Am J Ophthalmol 1988;105:419–420
20. Zierhut M, Kreissig F, Pickert A. Panuveitis with positive serological tests for syphilis and Lyme disease. J Clin Neuro Ophthalmol 1989;9:71–75
21. Lang GE, Schonherr U, Naumann GOH. Retinal vasculitis with proliferative retinopathy in a patient with evidence of *Borrelia burgdorferi* infection. Am J Ophthalmol 1991;111:243–244

22. Lightman DA, Brod RD. Branch retinal artery occlusion associated with Lyme disease. Arch Ophthalmol 1991;109:1198–1199
23. Orlin SE, Lauffer JL. Lyme disease keratitis. Am J Ophthalmol 1989;107:678–680
24. DeLuise VP, O'Leary MJ. Peripheral ulcerative keratitis related to Lyme disease. Am J Ophthalmol 1991;111:244–245
25. Eichenfield AH, Athreya BH. Lyme disease: of ticks and titers. J Pediatr 1989; 114:328–333
26. Schwartz BS, Goldstein MO, Ribeiro JMC, et al. Antibody testing in Lyme disease. A comparison of results in four laboratories. JAMA 1989;262:3431–3434
27. Lawton Smith J, Parsons TM, Paris-Hamelin AJ, Porschen RK. The prevalence of Lyme disease in a non-endemic area. A comparative serologic study in a south Florida eye clinic population. J Clin Neuro Ophthalmol 1989;9:148–155
28. Berg D, Abson KG, Prose NS. The laboratory diagnosis of Lyme disease. Arch Dermatol 1991;127:866–870
29. Winward KE, Lawton Smith J. Ocular disease in Caribbean patients with serologic evidence of Lyme borreliosis. J Clin Neuro Ophthalmol 1989;9:65–70
30. Lawton Smith J. Lyme disease appears to have many ocular manifestations. Arch Ophthalmol 1990;108:337
31. Wormser GP. Lyme disease. In: Platt R, ed. Current therapy in infectious diseases. Philadelphia: BC Decker, 1990:345–350

Contact Lens–related Infectious Keratitis

Millicent L. Palmer, M.D.

Robert A. Hyndiuk, M.D.

Infectious or microbial keratitis is an infection of the cornea characterized by an ulceration of the corneal epithelium associated with an underlying inflammatory infiltrate of the corneal stroma. Infectious keratitis is the most serious complication of contact lens wear. Complications of infectious keratitis include sight-threatening scar formation, scleral involvement, corneal perforation, and even loss of the eye.

The majority of contact lens users in the United States wear soft hydrogel lenses for cosmetic, refractive purposes. A 1990 survey conducted by the Contact Lens Council [1] revealed that approximately 25 million people in the United States, or 10% of the population, wear contact lenses. Sixty-six percent of contact lens wearers are female and 34% are male. The majority of contact lens users are in the 18- to 39-year age group: 31.5% aged 18 to 25 and 37.3% aged 26 to 39. Contact Lens Council marketing data for 1991 indicated that soft contact lenses (SCLs) accounted for 85% of the contact lens market, rigid gas-permeable lenses (RGPLs) 14%, and hard (polymethylmethacrylate [PMMA]) lenses 1%. In 1991, total contact lens retail sales in the United States amounted to $1,188,980,000 [1].

Contact lens wear is the most common predisposing factor for infectious keratitis in patients with previously healthy eyes [2]. Frequent reports of contact lens–associated infectious keratitis have been cited in the ophthalmic literature in the last 10 to 15 years [3–18]. With new developments in contact lens technology, reports of contact lens–associated ulcers have also been reported in wearers of disposable SCLs [19–26], high-Dk, extended-wear RGPLs [27], and planotinted contact lenses [28]. Although it is evident that all contact lens wearers are at risk, users of extended-

Article revised and updated from *Current Opinion in Infectious Diseases* 3:542–548, 1990, with permission from Current Science, Philadelphia, PA.

wear soft contact lenses (EWSCLs) are at particular risk [5, 8, 15, 18, 29–37].

The most important pathogens in contact lens–associated corneal infections are *Pseudomonas aeruginosa* [3–18, 20, 29, 38, 39] and *Acanthamoeba* species [38–60]. Other pathogens include *Staphylococcus* species, *Streptococcus* species, enteric gram-negative organisms, and the mixed flora of the eyelids, conjunctiva, and adnexa [3, 8, 10, 16, 39, 60]. Gram-positive organisms such as staphylococci and streptococci are more commonly associated with corneal ulcers in patients wearing aphakic and therapeutic contact lenses [3, 8, 10, 16, 39, 60–65]. Although they have been described in contact lens wearers, infections due to fungi are relatively uncommon [3, 12, 64, 66–69].

This chapter will focus on the important causes of contact lens–related infections—namely, *Pseudomonas* and *Acanthamoeba* keratitis. New insights into the epidemiological features, risk factors, and pathogenesis will be reviewed. Issues regarding prevention also will be highlighted.

■ Epidemiological Features and Risk Factors

The number of contact lens wearers has increased dramatically in the last decade. This has been paralleled by an increase in contact lens–associated ulcerative keratitis. It is unclear whether this fact represents an increase in rate of disease or a growing population at risk [70]. Historical perspectives and the importance of prospective clinical studies to evaluate important issues regarding long-term safety of contact lens wear, particularly the vision-threatening complication of infectious keratitis, have recently been addressed [71]. The growing popularity of contact lenses is largely attributable to their cosmetic and optical advantages. Many patients prefer EWSCLs to daily-wear soft contact lenses (DWSCLs) because of the added convenience. In 1980, the U.S. Food and Drug Administration (FDA) approved EWSCL wear for 30-day continuous (day and night) use and, by 1987, there were 4 million EWSCL users [71]. More recently, RGP and disposable SCLs have been made available for extended-wear use. Since approximately 1983, case reports and small clinical series have implied that users of EWSCLs were at greater risk than users of DWSCLs or hard lenses [5, 10, 15, 30–35]. Not until 1989 did well-designed prospective studies document the incidence and the relative risks of contact lens–related ulcerative keratitis [36, 37, 44].

A multicenter case-control study by Schein and colleagues [36] was the first statistical evaluation of the relative risk of ulcerative keratitis among users of DWSCLs and EWSCLs. It was concluded that overnight wear is the greatest risk factor for ulcerative keratitis in contact lens users. When compared to strict daily lens use, overnight wear increased the risk 10 to 15 times in EWSCL users and 9 times in occasional overnight DWSCL users. It was also noted that each consecutive day of lens use before cleaning EWSCLs increased the risk by at least 5%. Preexisting systemic disease was found to be associated with risk only in diabetics who wore DWSCLs. Interestingly, smoking was statistically associated with an increased risk in EWSCL users.

Poggio and co-workers [37] conducted a prospective study to assess the incidence of ulcerative keratitis among DWSCL and EWSCL users. The annual incidence of ulcerative keratitis, given the current pattern of lens wear, was estimated to be 4.1 per 10,000 DWSCL users (without overnight wear) and 20.9 per 10,000 EWSCL users. The lowest incidence was noted in wearers of hard (PMMA) lenses—2 per 10,000 annually. RGPL users had an incidence of 4.0 per 10,000. Of the hygiene-related practices, the most unfavorable effect was attributable to a dirty lens case.

Recent reports have documented the risk of ulcerative keratitis in wearers of disposable SCLs [19–26]. A recent case-control study compared the relative risk of ulcerative keratitis among disposable SCL users as compared to the risk among daily and extended-wear soft and gas-permeable lens users [24]. DWSCL users had the lowest risk of developing ulcerative keratitis and were assigned a risk ratio of 1.0. Users of RGPLs had a relative risk ratio of 1.3, and users of EWSCLs, 6.3. Disposable SCL users had the highest relative risk of 19.4.

Acanthamoeba keratitis was first reported in 1973 [72]. Historically, this infection has been associated with penetrating corneal trauma and exposure to contaminated water [13, 44, 48, 72–74]. It was not until 1984 that the first case of *Acanthamoeba* keratitis was documented in a contact lens wearer [45]. The association of contaminated homemade saline, *Acanthamoeba* keratitis, and SCL wear was later documented in 1985 [46]. Five species have been recovered from corneal isolates: *A. polyphaga*, *A. castellani*, *A. culbertsoni*, *A. rhysodes*, and *A. hatchetti* [43].

An epidemiological study by Stehr-Green and colleagues [44] estimated the number of acanthamoebic keratitis cases in the United States and the proportion of cases associated with three major risk factors—corneal trauma, exposure to polluted water, and contact lens wear. Two hundred eight cases were identified, and a number of important conclusions were reached:

1. The incidence of acanthamoebic keratitis in the United States is much higher than anticipated from published case reports, and contact lens wear is the predominant risk factor (85% of patients).
2. Although *Acanthamoeba* organisms are believed to be ubiquitous in nature, case reports were clustered in California, Texas, Florida, and Pennsylvania.
3. The median age was 29 years (range, 13 to 82 years).
4. There was no sex predilection noted.

Several risk factors for *Acanthamoeba* keratitis in SCL wearers were identified in a prospective study [73]. The use of homemade saline (for lens storage and postdisinfection rinsing), disinfecting lenses less frequently than manufacturers' recommendations, and wearing lenses while swimming were all associated with acanthamoebic keratitis. Use of hot tubs while wearing SCLs has also been identified as a risk factor [45].

■ Pathogenesis

Adhesion and entry are initial events and key prerequisites for the promotion of infectious keratitis [60]. An epithelial defect or stromal injury facilitates this process [75–78]. In EWSCL wearers, epithelial injury may occur in several ways: (1) Minor trauma may occur during lens insertion and removal; (2) toxins produced by adherent bacteria may be locally traumatic to the epithelium; and (3) large deposits on the lens may cause direct trauma to the epithelium, in addition to which a lens heavily coated with mucin or other debris may have reduced oxygen transmissibility, resulting in hypoxic stress [79]. The role of adherence of microorganisms to the contact lens and to the corneal epithelium and the importance of microbial contamination of contact lens care systems in the pathogenesis of contact lens-related corneal ulcers is summarized in Figures 1 and 2 and is discussed in more detail below.

Adherence to the Lens

Adherence of microorganisms, such as *Pseudomonas*, to the hydrophilic matrix of SCLs may play a key role in the pathogenesis of contact lens–related ulcers. In vitro studies have demonstrated the role of a polysaccharide biofilm in the adherence of *P. aeruginosa* and *Staphylococcus epidermidis* to the surface of EWSCLs [80]. This interaction between the biomaterial and bacterial organisms represents a self-protective environment for the propagation and inoculation of the organism [80]. The ability of *P. aeruginosa* to produce this slime envelope or biofilm has important implications in the pathogenesis of contact lens–related corneal ulcers.

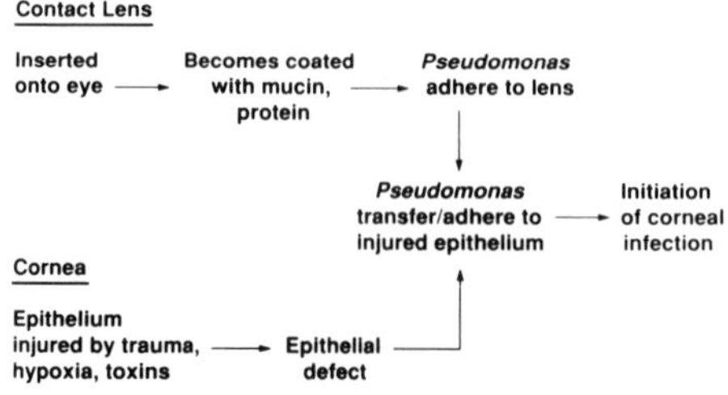

Figure 1 *Possible pathogenesis of* Pseudomonas *keratitis in contact lens wearers. (Adapted with permission from G. A. Stern. Prevention of contact lens-associated bacterial corneal ulcers. In: Friedlaender MH, ed. Prevention of eye diseases. New York: Mary Ann Liebert, Inc., 1988:123–130.)*

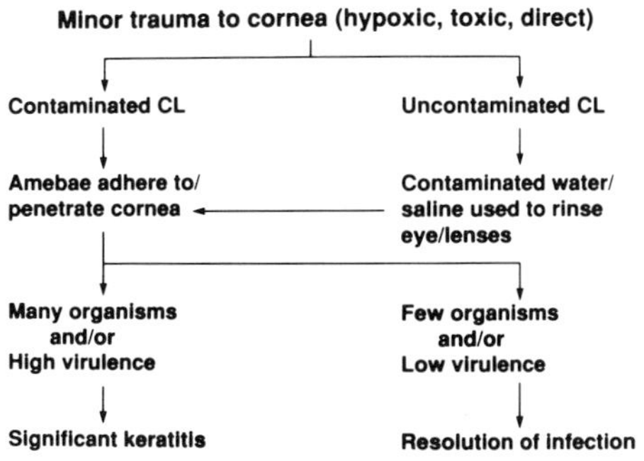

Minor trauma to cornea (hypoxic, toxic, direct)

Contaminated CL → Amebae adhere to/ penetrate cornea → Many organisms and/or High virulence → Significant keratitis

Uncontaminated CL → Contaminated water/ saline used to rinse eye/lenses → Few organisms and/or Low virulence → Resolution of infection

Figure 2 *Presumed pathogenesis of* Acanthamoeba *keratitis in contact lens wearers. (Adapted with permission from M. B. Moore, ed.* Acanthamoeba *keratitis in contact lens wearer: the patient is at fault. Cornea 1990;9[suppl 1]:S33–S35.)*

P. aeruginosa has been shown to adhere avidly to new [81] and worn [82, 83] SCLs. Contact lens coatings have also been implicated in facilitating bacterial adherence. More than 90% of the lens surface may become coated with tear film constituents (proteins, mucin, lipids, calcium) and, occasionally, microorganisms within 24 hours [84]. A propensity of bacteria to adhere to SCLs in areas of contact lens deposits has been noted by some authors [85–88]. Stern and Zam [85] demonstrated that *P. aeruginosa* can adhere to unworn SCLs but that adherence was enhanced 12-fold when the lens was coated with mucin or a combination of mucin and protein. It has been postulated that the increased incidence of *Pseudomonas* corneal ulcers in EWSCL wearers may be related to the heavy coating of mucin and tear film constituents facilitating adherence of the organism [79]. Adherent microorganisms on the contact lens may serve as a reservoir of potential pathogenic bacteria [40]. John and colleagues [89] demonstrated that bacterial adherence to hydrophilic SCLs was greater in viable *P. aeruginosa* than in organisms altered by heat or 3% hydrogen peroxide, proving that this is an active process. Effective enzymatic cleaning of mucin-coated hydrogel lenses has been shown to reduce adherence of *Pseudomonas* organisms to the lens [79]. However, electron-microscopical studies have shown that contact lens coatings on worn SCLs are not completely removed with surfactant or enzymatic cleaners [90]. Firm adherence of *Acanthamoeba* cysts and trophozoites to SCLs has also been demonstrated [91].

Adherence to Corneal Epithelium

P. aeruginosa has been shown in vitro to adhere more avidly than other bacterial species to corneal epithelial cells [92]. A well-designed experimental keratitis model demonstrated that *P. aeruginosa* adheres to and penetrates damaged corneal epithelium and stroma [75]. This has been confirmed by other investigators as well [93–98]. The transfer of organisms from contact lens to the cornea occurs through an interaction between the bacterial and corneal epithelial cell membranes [40, 93, 97].

Adult rabbit models of contact lens–related *Pseudomonas* keratitis revealed that infection developed only in traumatized corneas [99, 100]. The work of DiGaetano and co-workers [99] demonstrated that infectious keratitis was more common with mucin-coated, contaminated SCLs than with noncoated, contaminated lenses. In an EWSCL model, *Pseudomonas* keratitis developed without trauma [101, 102].

An intact corneal epithelium, with few exceptions, is an excellent barrier against microbial invasion [76]. However, the morphological study by Campbell and colleagues [103] revealed that *Acanthamoeba* trophozoites and cysts adhere equally well to intact corneal epithelium and bare Bowman's layer.

Microbial Contamination of Contact Lens Care Systems

Contamination of contact lens care systems has been identified as a source of pathogens in contact lens–associated infectious keratitis [31, 37, 46, 51, 57, 73, 104–109]. Donzis and co-workers [104] identified microbial contamination of contact lens care systems in 52 of 100 asymptomatic hard and soft lens wearers. This study also revealed that unpreserved saline solutions were consistently contaminated within 2 weeks of opening the cap. No contamination was noted in preserved solutions opened and used for less than 21 days. All homemade saline solution containers tested were contaminated. *Bacillus* species that produce spores resistant to heat and chemical disinfection systems were found in 7 patients. Heat-resistant endotoxin was detected in 26% of those tested.

Bacillus subtilis and *B. cereus* corneal ulcers associated with contamination of lens care systems have been described [105]. Chemical, oxidative (3% H_2O_2), and heat disinfection of the isolated organisms was compared against that for *S. epidermidis*. Only prolonged exposure (5 hours) of 3% H_2O_2 effectively eradicated both *Bacillus* species. Heat-resistant spores that survived five cycles of heat disinfection were noted. Therefore, once a lens care system is contaminated with *Bacillus* species, it may be almost impossible to eradicate the organism with recommended lens care regimens.

A follow-up study by the same authors documented that *Acanthamoeba* organisms were never isolated from lens care systems without coexisting bacteria or fungi. Thus, these coexistent species may be important for the survival and growth of *Acanthamoeba* [106].

Contamination of homemade saline solutions has been identified as a risk factor for *Acanthamoeba* keratitis [73]. The viability of acanthamoebic cysts from three species in ophthalmic saline, surfactant detergent cleaners, and chemical disinfecting solutions was assessed by Brandt and associates [110]. Hydrogen peroxide disinfectants were more effective than other disinfecting solutions in killing cysts. Disinfectants with thimerosal alone were less effective. However, cysts were detected for at least 6 hours after exposure in all disinfectant solutions. This time period exceeds the current manufacturers' recommendations. Saline solutions (viability 14 to 90 days) and daily cleaners (viability 1 to 90 days) were not effective in killing *Acanthamoeba* cysts. Heat disinfection (80°C for 10 minutes) is superior to chemical or oxidative disinfection systems [111].

■ Clinical and Diagnostic Features

General Findings

Patients usually present with symptoms of progressive discomfort, limbal or conjunctival hyperemia, photophobia, mucopurulent exudate, and variably decreased vision. Contact lens wearers frequently present with these symptoms and are found to have a corneal abrasion. Patching, even with an antibiotic, should be avoided because this may have an incubator effect, thus promoting an early corneal ulcer [4, 38].

The clinical hallmark of untreated microbial keratitis is a suppurative stromal infiltrate characterized by a dense yellow-white or gray-white infiltrate with an overlying epithelial defect on slit-lamp biomicroscopy. Stromal ulceration as well as pseudoguttae, stromal edema, and striae may be present.

Sterile corneal infiltrates in contact lens users, on the other hand, are typically small, relatively indolent, and focal or multifocal in distribution. These infiltrates often will resolve spontaneously after cessation of contact lens wear. The eye tends to be quieter in appearance, and the corneal tear film is usually acellular. The overlying epithelium usually is intact but punctate epithelial erosions may be observed [112, 113]. The differential diagnostic features of sterile versus infectious corneal infiltrates in contact lens wearers are summarized in Table 1 [112].

As a general rule, stromal infiltrates with an overlying epithelial defect should be considered infectious until proved otherwise. It is important to note that the degree of anterior chamber reaction may not be a reliable sign since contact lens wear alone may result in hypopyon formation [112].

Pseudomonas *Keratitis*

Corneal ulcers due to *P. aeruginosa* may be associated with severe pain. Unlike *Acanthamoeba* keratitis, *Pseudomonas* keratitis is a rapidly progressive suppurative process. Extensive ulceration and hypopyon are common. The involved corneal stroma is necrotic, and the surrounding stroma is classically edematous and gray with a ground-glass appearance (Fig 3). An immune ring (Wessely ring) infiltrate may also be observed. The immune ring observed in gram-negative ulcers such as those due to *Pseudomonas* is a result of the lipopolysaccharide endotoxin that is released when the

Table 1 *Clinical Comparisons between Sterile Infiltrate and Infectious Keratitis Associated with Contact Lens Wear*

Feature	Sterile infiltrate	Microbial keratitis
Onset	Subacute or acute; may occur soon after lens fitting or much later	Usually acute, although fungal and amebic keratitis may be slowly progressive
Incidence	Relatively common (approximately 5%)	Relatively uncommon (probably <1%)
Contact lens type	Any, but more common with soft hydrophilic and silicone lenses	Any, but more common with extended-wear soft lenses
Symptoms	Usually mild discomfort or foreign-body sensation	Increasing pain, both sharp and aching
Conjunctiva	Mild hyperemia with minimal discharge	Diffuse conjunctival injection with ciliary flush, eyelid edema and erythema, and mucopurulent discharge
Corneal epithelium	Usually intact or with punctate erosions	Usually ulcerated
Corneal stroma	White-gray focal or multifocal superficial stromal infiltrate with predilection for peripheral cornea	Yellow-white, suppurative infiltrate with blurred margins and surrounding inflammatory cells, frequently with mild stromal edema or striae; apparent predilection for central and superior cornea
Corneal endothelium	Minimal changes	Pseudoguttae with some Descemet's folds; occasionally has inflammatory plaque underlying stromal infiltrate
Anterior chamber	Clear or with minimal flare and cells; hypopyon may occur with or without stromal infiltrate	Miminal to marked iritis, occasionally with hypopyon

Source: Adapted with permission from [112].

organism dies [114]. This ring consists of polymorphonuclear leukocytes within the corneal stroma that are attracted by the alternate complement pathway and chemotaxis through properdin activation [114]. These ring infiltrates are believed to result from antigen-antibody precipitates [60, 114–116]. Descemetocele formation is usually indicative of imminent perforation.

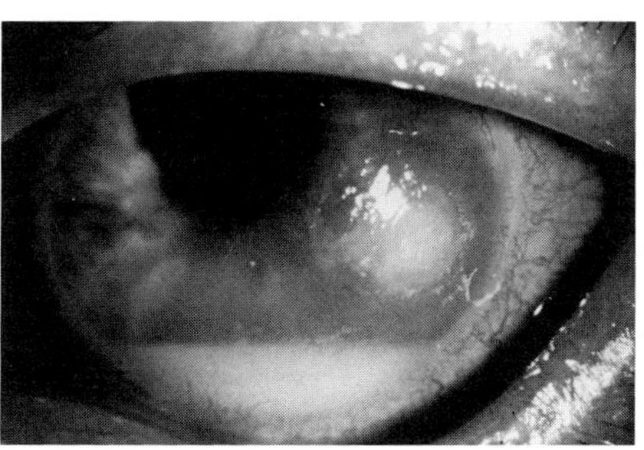

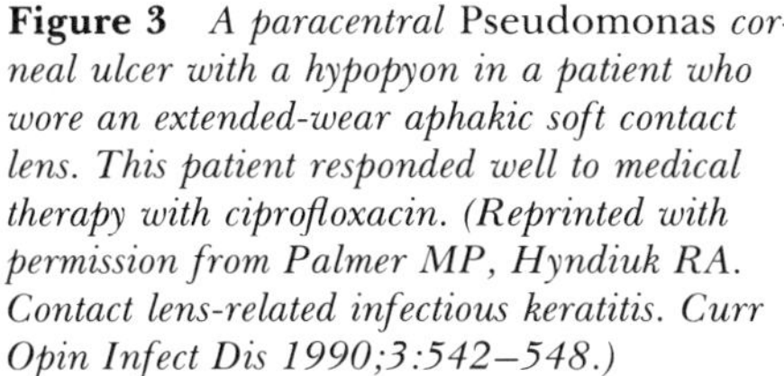

Figure 3   *A paracentral* Pseudomonas *corneal ulcer with a hypopyon in a patient who wore an extended-wear aphakic soft contact lens. This patient responded well to medical therapy with ciprofloxacin. (Reprinted with permission from Palmer MP, Hyndiuk RA. Contact lens-related infectious keratitis. Curr Opin Infect Dis 1990;3:542–548.)*

Acanthamoeba *Keratitis*

Acanthamoeba keratitis is an insidious, chronic, and progressive process. Severe pain that may be out of proportion to objective findings is a common presenting complaint. A dendritiform pattern of epithelial keratitis or disciform keratitis has been described in cases of early *Acanthamoeba* keratitis, leading to the misdiagnosis of herpes simplex virus (HSV) keratitis [11, 46, 48, 50, 58, 117–121]. Recurrent epithelial breakdown and healing is common [9, 38, 54, 56, 121] (Fig 4B). A ring-shaped infiltrate, partial or complete, may also be observed [13] (Fig 4A); however, it may be a relatively late sign [13]. Radial keratoneuritis has also been described [11] and has been postulated to explain the intense pain and diminished corneal sensation [121]. Descemetocele formation and perforation may be late sequelae.

An anterior nodular scleritis associated with extensive scleral ectasia in *Acanthamoeba* keratitis was recently described by Lindquist and colleagues [122]. The authors postulate that this may be due to a secondary immunological response to killed, necrotic organisms.

The diagnosis of *Acanthamoeba* keratitis should be suspected in any contact lens wearer, any case of therapeutically resistant stromal keratitis [48], and when routine cultures (aerobic and anaerobic) are nondiagnostic. Furthermore, *Acanthamoeba* keratitis should be included in the differential diagnosis of ring infiltrates, HSV keratitis, and even atypical corneal graft rejection [123]. Symptoms and signs of *Acanthamoeba* keratitis are summarized in Table 2 [120].

■ **Laboratory Evaluation**

It is imperative that corneal scrapings for smears and culture be obtained prior to initiation of antimicrobial therapy for infectious keratitis. Specimens should be directly inoculated onto standard media—blood, chocolate, and Sabouraud's dextrose agar and thioglycolate broth. Giemsa- and Gram-stained smears of corneal scrapings will aid in the identification

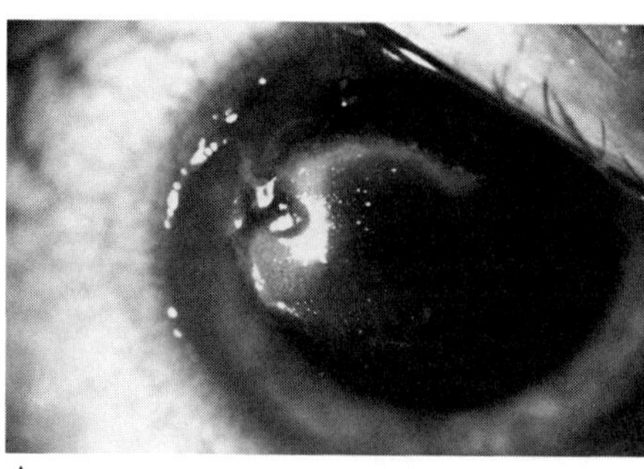
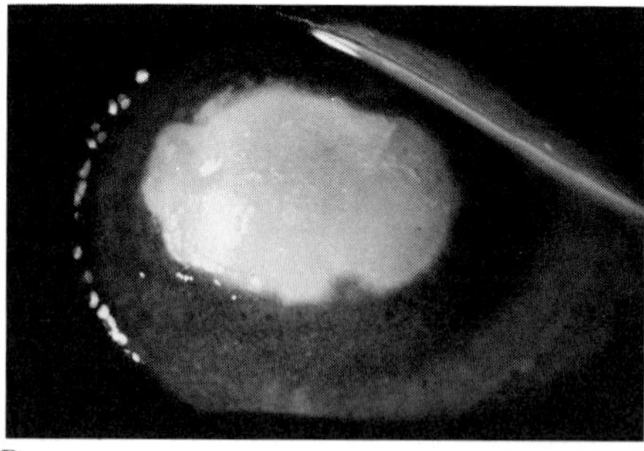

A   B

Figure 4 *(A)* Acanthamoeba *keratitis associated with a crescentic or partial ring infiltrate in a 19-year-old daily-wear soft contact lens wearer who used only unpreserved saline solution for lens soaking and storage. Her contact lens care system was contaminated with* Proteus, *Pseudomonas,* and Acanthamoeba *organisms. (B)* Acanthamoeba *keratitis in the same patient, demonstrating the large central overlying epithelial defect.*

of pathogens such as *Pseudomonas* and *Acanthamoeba* as well as fungal elements. In contact lens wearers, culturing lens care solutions and the contact lens case may be helpful in establishing the diagnosis [14, 18, 42, 46, 104–109].

Although *Acanthamoeba* cysts and trophozoites obtained from corneal scrapings stain with Gram stain, better results have been noted with Hemacolor (a fast Giemsa-Wright mixture; Harleco, Division of EM Industries, Inc., Gibbstown, NJ) as well as with Giemsa, trichrome, periodic acid–Schiff (PAS), Gomori methenamine silver (GMS), and Heidenhain's iron hematoxylin and eosin stain [13]. Calcofluor white (Polysciences, Inc., Warrington, PA), a chemofluorescent vital stain, is useful on corneal smears, frozen sections, vitrectomy specimens, and fixed tissue [118, 124]. It binds to chitin and cellulose in the cell walls of fungi and *Acanthamoeba* cysts [124]. Yeast, fungal elements, and *Acanthamoeba* cysts show bright apple-green fluorescence against a reddish-orange background [124]. An indirect immunofluorescent staining technique [45, 57, 120, 125, 126] and fluorescein-conjugated lectins [127] may also be used for *Acanthamoeba* species identification, but these techniques require a fluorescent microscope for visualization.

It is difficult to recover *Acanthamoeba* organisms by standard culture methods due to the biphasic cyst and trophozoite forms. Several techniques will facilitate identification. Corneal scrapings inoculated on a nonnutrient agar with an overlay of *Escherichia coli* or other gram-negative organisms [126] enhances recovery. The presence of *Acanthamoeba* trophozoites is indicated by a snail-tract clearing through the layer of bacteria. When direct inoculation is not possible, an ameba saline transport media and filter-culture technique may be utilized [128].

Histopathological examination of corneal specimens (corneal biopsy or

Table 2 *Symptoms and Signs of* Acanthamoeba *Keratitis*

	Stage of disease		
	Early (1–2 wk)	Moderately advanced (1–3 mo)	Advanced (3–6 mo)
Symptoms	Ocular hyperemia (red eye), no discharge, severe red pain	Ocular hyperemia (red eye), no discharge	Ocular hyperemia (red eye), no discharge, severe eye pain
Signs			
Eyelid	Reactive ptosis	Ptosis	Ptosis
Conjunctiva	Hyperemia	Hyperemia, chemosis, nodules	Hyperemia, chemosis, nodules, episcleritis
Sclera	—	—	Scleritis, nodules
Cornea			
Epithelium	Vesicular epithelium, pseudodendrite	Recurrent erosions, epithelial defects	Recurrent erosions, persistent defects
Subepithelial region	Small, white infiltrates	—	—
Stroma	Large, patchy, gray-white anterior and midstromal infiltrates	Ring infiltrate, single or double satellite infiltrates, central abscess	Ring abscess, central abscess, stromal liquefaction, sloughing, descemetocele, perforation, peripheral gutter, thinning, vascularization
Nerves	Single or multiple infiltrates	Single or multiple infiltrates	—
Anterior chamber	Rare cells and minimal flare	Moderate cell and flare	Hypopyon
Other	—	Preauricular node	Preauricular node

Source: Adapted with permission from [121].

transplant) may aid in making the diagnosis of microbial keratitis. Suggested special stains include Brown-Brenn or Brown-Hopps, tissue Gram stains, GMS, PAS, Luxol fast blue, and calcofluor white [124, 129].

■ Medical Treatment

Antimicrobial Agents

The initial treatment of microbial keratitis traditionally has been broad-spectrum fortified antibiotic drops. Frequent topical tobramycin or gentamicin and cefazolin or cefamandole may be initiated as soon as appropriate smears and cultures have been obtained. For the last 2 years, one of us (RAH) has used frequent ciprofloxacin (0.3% ciloxan) alone as the initial therapy in all suspected bacterial ulcers. Antibiotic loading doses of two drops every 5 minutes for five doses, followed by initial administration every 15 to 30 minutes, is advocated.

Ciprofloxacin is a new fluoroquinolone antibiotic with excellent broad-spectrum bactericidal activity against significant gram-positive and gram-negative pathogens that has recently received market approval for use in bacterial keratitis [130–135]. Variable sensitivity to streptococcal species has been described with systemic therapy [130, 131, 136, 137]. However, we have had excellent clinical results with topical therapy, including a case of infectious crystalline keratopathy due to alpha-hemolytic streptococci. Ciprofloxacin has excellent activity against *Pseudomonas* species with a minimum inhibitory concentration against 90% of all bacterial strains tested (MIC_{90}) value in the range of 0.12 to 1.0 [130]. Ocular penetration has also been excellent [138].

In vitro studies have demonstrated that the potency of ofloxacin and norfloxacin (chibroxin 0.3%) were equally or more effective than commercially available topical antibiotics against *P. aeruginosa* [137]. Ofloxacin was superior to norfloxacin, gentamicin, tobramycin, and chloramphenicol against *Staphylococcus* and *Streptococcus* species [137]. Ciprofloxacin as well as related fluoroquinolones hold great promise in our armamentarium for the treatment of bacterial keratitis, including in contact lens wearers. Further clinical trials are ongoing. A more detailed discussion of fluoroquinolones is presented in the chapter, "Role of the Fluoroquinolones in Ophthalmology."

Mills and co-workers [135] recently examined the efficacy of topical ceftazidime, a third-generation cephalosporin, in experimental bacterial keratitis. This, the most potent of the third-generation cephalosporins against *P. aeruginosa* and other *Pseudomonas* species, is less active against *S. aureus* but more stable to beta-lactamases than are cefotaxime and ceftizoxime. Ceftazidime may prove useful as monotherapy or in combination with an aminoglycoside in the treatment of bacterial keratitis.

Topical fortified antibiotic therapy has been the conventional means of drug delivery for microbial keratitis. Many other methods of drug delivery have been studied to enhance antibiotic bioavailability, ocular penetration, and efficacy [139]. Several reports evaluated collagen shields for the delivery of antibiotic agents [140–145]. A recent study by Silbiger and Stern [140] evaluated the efficacy of collagen shield delivery of gentamicin over a 24-hour period in experimentally induced *Pseudomonas* keratitis. The use of antibiotic-impregnated collagen shields augmented with topical therapy was more effective than topical therapy alone. This concurs with the results of Sawusch and co-workers [141]. However, topical antibiotic therapy every 30 minutes was superior to collagen shields supplemented with topical therapy every 3 hours. The authors recognized that the use of antibiotic-impregnated collagen shields supplemented with more frequent topical therapy, perhaps every 1 to 2 hours, may have been equivalent to topical therapy every 30 minutes. However, then one may argue that the increased cost of collagen shields would not be justified by only a slight increase in the convenience of drug administration. The authors conclude that the use of collagen shields as an antibiotic drug delivery device should not replace the gold standard of frequent topical fortified antibiotics before further clinical trials with antibiotic-impregnated collagen shields are undertaken.

Subconjunctival antibiotic administration may be indicated for severe deep ulcers and if fortified topical drops are not available [60]. Other indications for concurrent subconjunctival administration include corneal ulcers associated with endophthalmitis, scleral extension, or imminent perforation [60].

The topical antibiotic regimen is modified after 24 to 48 hours based on the clinical response and culture results. Further modifications in treatment are made on the basis of antibiotic sensitivity testing. Fortified drops should be continued until the cornea has reepithelialized and then should be gradually tapered depending on the clinical response. Once nocturnal dosing is tapered or discontinued, bedtime and morning loading doses to maximize antibiotic corneal concentrations is recommended.

Acanthamoeba *Keratitis*

The treatment of *Acanthamoeba* keratitis remains a challenging problem. Difficulty in eradicating this infection is related to the biphasic (cyst and trophozoite) nature of the organism [38], the often advanced stage of infection at the time of diagnosis, and the variable virulence of different strains [56]. Medical cures have, however, been reported [54–56, 146, 147]. The currently recommended therapy for *Acanthamoeba* keratitis includes topical propamidine isethionate (Brolene), dibromopropamidine 0.15% (Brolene ointment), neomycin–polymyxin B–gramicidin (Neosporin), and miconazole (Monistat) or clotrimazole (Lotrimin) in conjunction with oral ketoconazole (Nizoral) [46, 52, 54–56, 58]. Oral itraconazole has also been used [148]. Systemic ketaconazole should be given in a single daily dose of 200 to 600 mg [121]. Liver function tests must be followed weekly while using this drug. In general, prolonged medical therapy for *Acanthamoeba* keratitis usually is necessary.

Pentamidine isethionate (Pentam 300), a parenteral antiprotozoal agent used in the treatment of *Pneumocystis carinii* pneumonia in patients with the acquired immunodeficiency syndrome (AIDS), can be formulated from the intravenous powder (0.05 to 0.1%) for topical use pending the availability of Brolene [121]. Although efficacious in the treatment of *Acanthamoeba* keratitis, pentamidine has greater ocular toxicity [121].

■ Adjuvant Therapy

Medical Therapy

Cycloplegics such as 5% homatropine, 0.25% scopolamine, or 1% atropine are used routinely. These agents reduce pain from ciliary spasm and aid in the prevention of synechiae formation.

Corticosteroids alter the host immunological responses to infection, and therefore their role in infectious keratitis has been controversial [149–154]. Studies have demonstrated that concurrent corticosteroids do not inhibit drug efficacy [149] or enhance bacterial replication [150] when used with adequate anti–microbial therapy. However, *P. aeruginosa* replication in the cornea has been enhanced if antibiotic therapy is inadequate [151, 153]. Therefore, it is important to avoid use of corticosteroids early in the course prior to the availability of culture and sensitivity results. Delay in corneal sterilization and wound healing [153] and recurrence of *Pseudomonas* keratitis [154] has been observed. A controlled prospective trial by Carmichael and associates [155] compared antibiotic therapy with and without corticosteroids in bacterial keratitis and found no difference in visual outcome. Corticosteroids are contraindicated in eyes with advanced thinning, in which perforation is a threat.

The effects of adjunctive corticosteroids in the medical management of *Acanthamoeba* keratitis have been equivocal. Delay in diagnosis and treatment with topical corticosteroids prior to initiation of appropriate antiamebic therapy are common confounding variables in reported cases [56]. Although the effect of corticosteroids on the organism's morphogenesis (from cyst to trophozoite and vice versa) is not fully understood, Osata and colleagues [156] reported inhibition of morphogenesis by dexamethasone in broth suspensions. It is the authors' contention that by preventing free transformation of the two forms of the organism, corticosteroids may allow amebicidal agents to destroy active trophozoites while host responses clear the cyst. However, no consistent clinical response to topical steroids has been observed in *Acanthamoeba* keratitis [56, 147]. In a study by Rabinovitch and co-workers [157] evaluating clinical signs of predictors of outcome, a multivariate analysis revealed that use of corticosteroids is the sole parameter in predicting medical failure. These investigators concluded that corticosteroids are contraindicated.

Sulindac (Clinoril), a nonsteroidal antiinflammatory agent, has been recommended in lieu of narcotic analgesics or retrobulbar alcohol blocks for pain management in patients with *Acanthamoeba* keratitis [51, 121]. In our clinical experience, it has also been useful for pain management in other forms of infectious keratitis. The recommended oral dose is 200 mg two [51] to four [121] times daily. Other nonsteroidal antiinflammatory agents have been used in the management of scleritis associated with *Acanthamoeba* keratitis [56].

Surgical Therapy

Debridement   Debridement of bacterial and acanthamoebic ulcers has been advocated on a routine basis by some authors [59, 60, 147, 148, 158]. This prevents early reepithelialization over areas of stromal infiltrates, facilitating antibiotic penetration, and removes proteinaceous and mucoid discharge that may bind antimicrobials. In addition, it may potentially remove microbial or antigen load. Debrided material may also provide a generous specimen for culture or reculture as indicated. Debridement can be accomplished using a Kimura spatula, cotton-tipped applicator, cellulose sponge, or calcium alginate swab. In a moderate or severe ulcer, we routinely debride daily any healing epithelium over an active infiltrate, using a cellulose sponge, until the infiltrate begins to resolve.

Tissue Adhesive   Cyanoacrylate medical-grade tissue glue may be useful for repair in cases of progressive corneal necrosis, in thin descemetoceles, or in small corneal perforations [159]. An inhibitory effect on the bacteria has also been noted [160]. The glue, however, is toxic to the corneal endothelium and lens and therefore should be utilized only in cases of small perforations, unless it is used with a free tissue patch [161].

Patch Grafts and Conjunctival Flaps   As an alternative to using tissue adhesives, a patch graft may be employed in cases of small perforations [114, 160]. Conjunctival flaps may also be used in peripheral ulcers to promote healing. They are rarely indicated, however, in cases of central ulceration except when associated with impaired epithelial healing. The results of using conjunctival flaps in *Acanthamoeba* keratitis have generally been poor; the flaps undergo necrosis and the underlying infection progresses [121].

Cryotherapy   Cryotherapy has been shown to have bactericidal effects in an experimental animal model of infectious keratitis [162]. It also has been known to play a role in the treatment of an occasional case of bacterial keratitis caused by gram-negative organisms [162]. However, this form of therapy causes damage to the corneal endothelium at the temperatures needed to destroy the organism and therefore should be limited to peripheral corneal ulcers, scleral ulcers, or abscesses that are not controlled with routine medical therapy.

Previous experimental and clinical reports have indicated unfavorable results with cryotherapy in *Acanthamoeba* keratitis [163]. This technique failed to kill *Acanthamoeba* cysts, and infected eyes did not tolerate the procedure well [121]. In 5 cases of medically unresponsive *Acanthamoeba* keratitis that underwent cryotherapy to the host cornea at the time of primary or repeat penetrating keratoplasty, a favorable outcome was achieved in 3 of 5 cases, but there was no conclusive evidence that this technique eliminated the organism [164]. Currently, cryotherapy in *Acanthamoeba* keratitis is not recommended since it may cause corneal vascularization, tissue necrosis, and increased inflammation [121].

Penetrating Keratoplasty   Penetrating keratoplasty may be necessary in infections that are not controlled medically, in thin or perforated corneas or, later, to rehabilitate optically a scarred cornea. Ideally, prior to surgical intervention, one should attempt to sterilize the cornea and reduce inflammation to a minimum. Intensive antibiotic therapy, along with topical or systemic steroids, should be employed immediately preoperatively. Even in the cases of perforation, it is advocated that the eye be treated with antibiotics for at least 24 hours before operation. A Hessburg-Barron vacuum trephine is often helpful in trephination of a soft eye. Adequate iridectomies, as well as an oversized graft, are strongly recommended. The excised corneal button should be submitted for histopathological study with special tissue stains to assess adequate surgical margins. A portion of the button should also be submitted for cultures and sensitivity testing to confirm the identity of the organism as well as its viability and sensitivity. This is important in guiding the clinician to appropriate antibiotic therapy postoperatively [129]. Penetrating keratoplasty is often necessary in cases of recalcitrant *Acanthamoeba* keratitis. A recurrent infection rate as high as 25% has been reported [38]. The timing of penetrating keratoplasty remains controversial. It is recommended that keratoplasty be deferred until the infection has been resolved by medical therapy or host defenses or until at least 1 year after onset [121].

■ Prevention

General Principles

The importance of preventive measures in microbial keratitis in contact lens wearers cannot be overemphasized. Careful history, patient selection, an optimal fitting relationship between contact lens and cornea, and patient compliance with contact lens–wearing schedules, hygienic regimens, and medical supervision are key factors. Patients who are unreliable and who have unrealistic expectations are poor contact lens candidates. In addition, individuals who work in unsuitable occupational environments in terms of hygiene should be discouraged from contact lens wear. Good personal hygiene is also important.

Patient education and reeducation in acceptable lens care practices by the contact lens practitioner should be a priority. Patients must be informed of important warning signs and symptoms—namely, pain, redness, and decreased vision—and must be cautioned to remove lenses promptly and seek an ophthalmologist's advice should any of these occur. It is imperative that contact lens wearers have a current spectacle correction in order to rest the eyes and to serve as a backup in the event of eye irritation or infection.

Patient Selection

Patient selection begins with medical, drug, social, and occupational histories. Abnormalities of eyelid position or mechanics, eyelid skin, lid margins, conjunctiva, and cornea must be identified.

Contact lens fitting in monocular patients should be avoided. Monocular patients should be visually rehabilitated with spectacle correction using polycarbonate safety lenses.

Evaluation of tear production is also important. *Dry eyes* is a general term used to describe a spectrum of entities resulting in disruption of ocular surface integrity [165–168]. This may involve aqueous tear deficiency, mucin deficiency, or tear film instability due to blepharitis (meibomian gland dysfunction) and primary epitheliopathy (such as reduced corneal sensation or corneal scars) [166]. Good tear exchange is necessary for normal ocular surface toileting. It is important to note that only 1% of tear film is exchanged with SCLs versus 14% with rigid lenses [40]. This may contribute to the greater incidence of infectious keratitis among SCL wearers.

Normal blinking (15 times per minute) plays a crucial role in the maintenance of adequate tear exchange. Poor blink habits may be associated with low-riding lens, 3 and 9 o'clock staining, corneal edema, contact lens deposit formation, contact lens intolerance and, ultimately, contact lens failure [167]. Blinking should be carefully observed, and contact lens wearers should be made aware of its significance.

These historical and objective findings will help the practitioner make rational decisions regarding contact lens selection, wearing schedules, and the frequency of patient follow-up.

Contact Lens Hygiene

Contact lens users must comply with the manufacturers' lens care guidelines, especially regarding disinfection. Disinfection of contact lenses refers to the probability that no harmful bacterial contaminants will be present when the contact lenses are returned to the patient's eye [169]. A detailed discussion of contact lens hygiene is beyond the scope of this chapter but has been reviewed in detail elsewhere [170–172]. Briefly, thermal, chemical, and oxidative disinfection regimens are the main types of disinfection systems. All forms of contact lens disinfection must be preceded by a cleaning step. Heat disinfection remains superior to chemical systems in eliminating *Acanthamoeba* cysts and trophozoites [111]. Prolonged use of nonpreserved saline lens care solutions should be avoided due to the known risk of contamination. Aerosolized saline or unit-dose vials are recommended. Homemade saline solution should be eliminated from lens care. The use of intravenous saline solution by health care workers should be discouraged. Patients must also be warned that tap water and distilled water are not sterile. Saline rinses should therefore be used for RGP lenses. Swimming and use of hot tubs while wearing contact lenses should be avoided. Moreover, hand washing must be emphasized as an important step before any contact lens manipulation.

Patients often inquire as to how to care for their contact lenses if they are not going to wear them for a period of time. Some authors [172] recommend that rigid lenses, as well as the lens case, be cleaned and the lenses stored dry. Soft lenses should be cleaned and chemically disinfected after removal and stored in the refrigerator on an interim basis. If the lenses are not worn during the week, they should again be disinfected, and every week thereafter if not worn. If heat disinfection is used on soft lenses, they should be cleaned thoroughly and disinfected at least once weekly. Interim storage in the refrigerator is again recommended. Furthermore, lenses should be cleaned and disinfected once more prior to resuming normal wear. Whether chemical, oxidative, or heat disinfection is used, it is important to note the expiration date on the solutions.

A clean lens case has been identified as conferring a protective effect against the risk of contact lens–related corneal ulcers [37]. Contact lens–soaking solution in the case must be replaced daily. Anecdotally, experienced contact lens practitioners have recommended immersing the contact lens case in boiling water and allowing it to air dry between contact lens wearing and storage. A recent study recommended microwaving the contact lens case [173]. Mechanical cleaning of the contact lens case with a mild soap (e.g., no-tears baby shampoo) using a cotton-tipped applicator, clean toothbrush, or pipe cleaner may be indicated to clean grooved or hard-to-reach surfaces. Frequent contact lens case replacement may be the best alternative.

Trial contact lenses used in the office carry a potential risk of transmitting infectious agents, including the human immunodeficiency virus [174]. Therefore, a number of precautions must be observed to ensure safety in the office. Heat disinfection of hydrogel lenses is sufficient to destroy all infectious agents that may be present in low-water-content SCLs. Medium-

or high-water-content lenses should be disinfected with a two-step hydrogen peroxide system [174–178]. The use of disposable lenses in trial fittings may eliminate this risk because such lenses are discarded and a new sterile lens is used for each patient.

The Centers for Disease Control recommend a hydrogen peroxide disinfecting system for trial rigid lenses [174–176]. A recent clinical alert from the American Academy of Ophthalmology indicates that solutions preserved with chlorhexidine preservative are also effective against a number of pathogens including the human immunodeficiency virus (HIV) [177]. This has been supported by a study by Vogt and colleagues [178], who show that surfactant cleaners containing chlorhexidine can eradicate HIV from both new soft and rigid lenses inoculated with the virus. The Centers for Disease Control, however, have not yet approved chlorhexidine for disinfection for HIV. It is recommended that rigid lenses be stored dry after disinfection.

Contact Lens–Wearing Schedule

The FDA has recently recommended a reduced wearing schedule of continuous or extended-wear soft contact lenses. The current recommendation is that contact lenses be worn for no more than 7 days of continuous wear, at which time the lenses should be removed, cleaned, and disinfected [179].

Disposable SCLs as well as frequent-replacement DWSCLs have recently been produced by several manufacturers. It is hoped that the replacement regimens associated with these lenses will promote improved ocular health as well as patient compliance and regular medical supervision.

■ Summary

Infectious keratitis is the most serious complication of contact lens use. Virtually all contact lens wearers are at risk. Initial therapy consists of frequent broad-spectrum fortified antibiotic drops after appropriate laboratory workup. *Pseudomonas* and *Acanthamoeba* species are the most important causes of contact lens–associated ulcers. *Acanthamoeba* keratitis produces significant ocular morbidity, and treatment is not always effective. Recent studies have provided new insights regarding the incidence, risk factors, and pathogenesis of contact lens–related infectious keratitis. Extended-wear soft contact lens wearers are at greatest risk. With our present understanding of the pathogenesis and risk factors of contact lens–related infectious keratitis, daily-wear schedules are strongly advised. Even under the best of lens care conditions, infectious keratitis may still occur. It is therefore imperative that patients be informed to remove their lenses and seek medical evaluation if any discomfort develops.

This work was supported in part by an unrestricted departmental grant from Research to Prevent Blindness, Inc., New York, NY, and by National Eye Institute core grant EY01931-15, Bethesda, MD.

■ References

1. Contact Lens Council survey 1990–1991, Washington, D.C.
2. Dart JKG. Predisposing factors in microbial keratitis: the significance of contact lens wear. Br J Ophthalmol 1988;72:926–930
3. Alfonso E, Mandelbaum S, Fox M, et al. Ulcerative keratitis associated with contact lens wear. Am J Ophthalmol 1986;101:429–433
4. Clemons CS, Cohen EJ, Arentsen JJ, et al. *Pseudomonas* ulcers following patching of corneal abrasions associated with contact lens wear. CLAO J 1987;13:161–164
5. Cohen EJ, Laibson PR, Arentsen JJ, et al. Corneal ulcers associated with cosmetic extended wear soft contact lenses. Ophthalmology 1987;94:109–114
6. Cohen EJ, Parlato CJ, Arentsen JJ, et al. Medical and surgical treatment of *Acanthamoeba* keratitis. Am J Ophthalmol 1987;94:109–114
7. Donnenfeld ED, Cohen EJ, Arentsen JJ, et al. Changing trends in contact lens associated corneal ulcers: an overview of 116 cases. CLAO J 1986;12:145–149
8. Galentine PG, Cohen EJ, Laibson PR, et al. Corneal ulcers associated with contact lens wear. Arch Ophthalmol 1984;102:891–894
9. Lindquist TD, Sher MA, Doughman DJ. Clinical signs and medical therapy of early *Acanthamoeba* keratitis. Arch Ophthalmol 1988;106:73–77
10. Mondino BJ, Weissman OD, Farb MD, et al. Corneal ulcers associated with daily wear and extended wear contact lens. Am J Ophthalmol 1986;102:58–65
11. Moore MB, McCulley JP, Kaufman HE, et al. Radial keratoneuritis as a presenting sign in *Acanthamoeba* keratitis. Ophthalmology 1986;93:1310–1315
12. Ormerod LD, Smith RE. Contact lens associated microbial keratitis. Arch Ophthalmol 1986;104:79–83
13. Theodore FH, Jakobiec FA, Jeuchter KB, et al. The diagnostic value of a ring infiltrate in *Acanthamoeba* keratitis. Ophthalmology 1985;92:1471–1479
14. Wilson LA, Schlitzer R, Ahern D. *Pseudomonas* corneal ulcers associated with soft contact lens wear. Am J Ophthalmol 1981;92:546–554
15. Chalupa E, Swarbrick HA, Holden BA, et al. Severe corneal infections associated with contact lens wear. Ophthalmology 1987;94:17–22
16. Laibson PR, Donnenfeld ED. Contact ulcers related to contact lens use. Int Ophthalmol Clin 1986;26:3–15
17. Krachmer JH, Purcell JJ. Bacterial corneal ulcers in cosmetic SCL wearers. Arch Ophthalmol 1978;96:57–61
18. Cooper RL, Constable IJ. Infective keratitis in soft contact lens wearers. Br J Ophthalmol 1977;61:250–254
19. Serdahl CL, Mannis MJ, Shapiro DR. Infiltrative keratitis associated with disposable soft contact lenses. Arch Ophthalmol 1989;107:322–323
20. Killingsworth DW, Stern GA. *Pseudomonas* keratitis associated with the use of disposable soft contact lenses. Arch Ophthalmol 1989;107:795–796
21. Dunn JP, Mondino BJ, Weissman BA, et al. Corneal ulcers associated with disposable hydrogel contact lenses. Am J Ophthalmol 1989;108:113–117

22. Ficker L, Hunter P, Seal D, Wright P. *Acanthamoeba* keratitis occurring with disposable contact lens wear. Am J Ophthalmol 1989;108:453
23. Goyal AK, Sulewski ME, Nichols CW. Corneal ulcers in disposable contact lens wearers. Invest Ophthalmol Vis Sci 1992(suppl);33(4):1209 (abstract)
24. Buehler PO, Schein OD, Stamler JF, Verdiek DV. Increased risk of ulcerative keratitis among disposable SCL users. Invest Ophthalmol Vis Sci 1992(suppl); 33(4):1209 (abstract)
25. Maguen E, Tsai JC, Martinez M, et al. A retrospective study of disposable extended-wear lenses in 100 patients. Ophthalmology 1991;98:1685–1689
26. Rajpal RK, Sperber LTD, Chien AM, et al. Recent trends, risk factors, and etiological agents in ulcerative keratitis. Invest Ophthalmol Vis Sci 1992(suppl);33(4):1209 (abstract)
27. Ehrlich M, Weissman BA, Mondino BJ. *Pseudomonas* corneal ulcer after use of extended-wear rigid gas-permeable contact lenses. Cornea 1989;8:225–226
28. Snyder RW, Brenner MB, Wiley L, et al. Microbial keratitis associated with plano tinted contact lenses. CLAO J 1991;17(4):252–255
29. Eichenbaum JW, Feldstein J, Podos SM. Extended-wear aphakic soft contact lenses and corneal ulcers. Br J Ophthalmol 1982;66:663–666
30. Weissman BA, Mondino BJ, Pettit TH, Hofbauer JD. Corneal ulcers associated with extended-wear soft contact lenses. Am J Ophthalmol 1984;97:476–481
31. Adams CP, Cohen EJ, Laibson PR, et al. Corneal ulcers in patients with cosmetic extended-wear contact lenses. Am J Ophthalmol 1983;96:705–709
32. Wilhelmus KR. Review of clinical experience with microbial keratitis associated with contact lens wear. CLAO J 1987;13:211–214
33. Hassman G, Sugar J. *Pseudomonas* corneal ulcer with extended-wear soft contact lenses for myopia. Arch Ophthalmol 1983;101:1549–1550
34. Lemp MA, Blackman HJ, Wilson LA, Leveille AS. Gram negative corneal ulcers in elderly aphakic eyes with extended-wear lenses. Ophthalmology 1984;91:60–63
35. Spoor TC, Hartel WC, Wyann P, Spoor DK. Complications of continuous-wear soft contact lenses in a nonreferral population. Arch Ophthalmol 1984;102: 1312–1313
36. Schein OD, Glynn RJ, Poggio EC, et al. The relative risk of ulcerative keratitis among users of daily-wear and extended-wear contact lenses. N Engl J Med 1989;321:773–778
37. Poggio EC, Glynn RJ, Schein OD, et al. The incidence of ulcerative keratitis among users of daily-wear and extended-wear contact lenses. Am J Ophthalmol 1989; 108:658–664
38. Bowden FW, Cohen EJ. Corneal ulcerations with contact lenses. Ophthalmol Clin North Am 1989;2:267–273
39. Schein OD, Omerod LD, Barraquer E, et al. Microbiology of contact lens–related keratitis. Cornea 1989;8(4):281–285
40. Stern MA. *Pseudomonas* keratitis and contact lens wear: the lens/eye at fault. Cornea 1990;9(suppl 1):S36–S38
41. Jones DB. *Acanthamoeba*—the ultimate opportunist. Am J Ophthalmol 1986;2: 527–530
42. *Acanthamoeba* keratitis associated with contact lenses—United States. MMWR 1986;35:405–408
43. *Acanthamoeba* keratitis in SCL wearers. MMWR 1987;36:397–404
44. Stehr-Green JK, Bailey TM, Visvesvara GS. The epidemiology of *Acanthamoeba* keratitis in the United States. Am J Ophthalmol 1989;107:331–336
45. Samples JR, Binder PS, Luibel FJ, et al. *Acanthamoeba* keratitis possibly acquired from a hot tub. Arch Ophthalmol 1984;102:707–710
46. Moore MB, McCulley JP, Luckenbach M, et al. *Acanthamoeba* keratitis associated with soft contact lenses. Am J Ophthalmol 1985;100:396–403

47. Blackman HJ, Rao NA, Lemp MA, Visvesvara GS. *Acanthamoeba* keratitis successfully treated with penetrating keratoplasty. Suggested immunogenic mechanism of action. Cornea 1984;3:125–130

48. Cohen EJ, Buchanan HW, Laughrea PA, et al. Diagnosis and management of *Acanthamoeba* keratitis. Am J Ophthalmol 1985;100:389–395

49. Wilhelmus KR, Osato MS, Font RL. Rapid diagnosis of *Acanthamoeba* keratitis using calcofluor white. Arch Ophthalmol 1986;104:1309–1312

50. Moore MB, McCulley JP, Newton C, et al. *Acanthamoeba* keratitis. A growing problem in soft and hard contact lens wearers. Ophthalmology 1987;94:1654–1661

51. Koenig SB, Solomon JM, Hyndiuk RA, et al. *Acanthamoeba* keratitis associated with gas permeable contact lens wear. Am J Ophthalmol 1987;103:832

52. Cohen EJ, Parloto CJ, Arentsen JJ, et al. Medical and surgical treatment of *Acanthamoeba* keratitis. Am J Ophthalmol 1987;103:615–625

53. Dornic DI, Wolf T, Dillon WH, et al. *Acanthamoeba* keratitis in soft contact lens wearers. J Am Optom Assoc 1987;58:482–486

54. Lindquist TD, Sher NA, Doughman DJ. Clinical signs and medical therapy of early *Acanthamoeba* keratitis. Arch Ophthalmol 1988;106:73–77

55. Moore MB, McCulley JP. *Acanthamoeba* keratitis associated with contact lenses: six consecutive cases of successful management. Br J Ophthalmol 1989;73:271–275

56. Auran JD, Starr MB, Jakobiec FA. *Acanthamoeba* keratitis: a review of the literature. Cornea 1987;6:2–26

57. Epstein RJ, Wilson LA, Visvesvara GS, Plounde EG. Rapid diagnosis of *Acanthamoeba* keratitis from corneal scrapings using indirect fluorescent antibody staining. Arch Ophthalmol 1986;104:1318–1321

58. Hirst LW, Green WR, Merz W, et al. Management of *Acanthamoeba* keratitis. A case report and review of the literature. Ophthalmology 1984;91:1105–1111

59. Holland GN, Donzis PB. Rapid resolution of early *Acanthamoeba* keratitis after epithelial debridement. Am J Ophthalmol 1987;104:87–88

60. Hyndiuk RA, Skorich DN, Burd EM. Bacterial keratitis. In: Tabbara KF, Hyndiuk RA, eds. Infections of the eye. Boston: Little, Brown, 1986:303–330

61. Milauskas AT. *Pseudomonas aeruginosa* contamination of hydrophilic contact lenses and solutions. Trans Am Acad Ophthalmol Otolaryngol 1972;76:511–516

62. Dohlman CH, Boruchoff SA, Mobilia EF. Complications in use of soft contact lenses in corneal disease. Arch Ophthalmol 1973;90:367–371

63. Dohlman CH. Complications in therapeutic soft lens wear. Trans Am Acad Ophthalmol Otolaryngol 1974;78:399–405

64. Brown SI, Bloomfield S, Pearce DB, Tragakis M. Infections with the therapeutic soft lens. Arch Ophthalmol 1974;91:275–277

65. Smith GS, Lindstrom RL, Nelson DJ, et al. Corneal ulcer-infiltrate associated with SCL use following PKP. Cornea 1984;3:131–134

66. Wilson LA, Ahearn DG. Association of fungi with extended-wear soft contact lenses. Am J Ophthalmol 1986;101:434–436

67. Yamamoto GK, Pavan-Langston D, Stowe GC, et al. Fungal invasion of a therapeutic SCL and cornea. Am J Ophthalmol 1979;11:1731–1735

68. Wilhelmus KR, Robinson NM, Font RA, et al. Fungal keratitis in contact lens wearers. Am J Ophthalmol 1988;106:708–714

69. Strelow SA, Kent HD, Eagle RC, Cohen ET. A case of contact lens–related *Fusarium solani* keratitis. CLAO J 1992;18:125–127

70. Schein O, Hibberd P, Kenyon JR. Contact lens complications: incidental or epidemic? Am J Ophthalmol 1987;102:116–117

71. Smith RE, MacRae SM. Contact lenses—convenience and complications. N Engl J Med 1989;321:824–826

72. Visvesvara GS. Free-living pathogenic amoeba. In: Lennette EH, Balows A, Hausler WJ Jr, eds. Manual of clinical microbiology, ed 3. Washington, DC: American Society for Microbiology, 1980:704–708

73. Stehr-Green JK, Bailey TM, Brandt FH, et al. *Acanthamoeba* keratitis in SCL wearers: a case-control study. JAMA 1987;258:57–60
74. Ma P, Willaert E, Juechter KB, et al. A case of keratitis due to *Acanthamoeba* in NY, NY, and features of 10 cases. J Infect Dis 1981;143:662–667
75. Hyndiuk RA. Experimental *Pseudomonas* keratitis. Trans Am Ophthalmol Soc 1981;79:541–624
76. Snyder RW, Hyndiuk RA. Mechanisms of bacterial invasion. In: Duane TD, Jaeger EA, eds. Biomedical foundations of ophthalmology, ed 2. Philadelphia: Lippincott, 1988:1–7
77. Hyndiuk RA, Snyder RW. Infectious diseases—bacterial keratitis. In: Smolin G, Thoft R, eds. The cornea, ed 2. Boston: Little, Brown, 1987;5:193–255
78. Hyndiuk RA, Seideman S. Clinical and laboratory techniques in external ocular disease and endophthalmitis. In: Fedukowitz HB, ed. External infections of the eye, ed 2. New York: Appleton-Century-Crofts, 1978:258–275
79. Stern GA, Zam ZS. The effect of enzymatic contact lens cleaning on adherence of *Pseudomonas aeruginosa* to SCL. Ophthalmology 1987;94:115–119
80. Slusher MM, Myrvik QN, Lewis JC, Gristina HG. Extended-wear lenses, biofilm and bacterial adhesion. Arch Ophthalmol 1987;105:110–115
81. Duran JA, Refojo MF, Gipson IK, Kenyon KR. *Pseudomonas* attachment to new hydrogel lenses. Arch Ophthalmol 1987;105:106–109
82. Butras SI, Klotz SA, Misra RP. The adherence of *Pseudomonas aeruginosa* to soft contact lenses. Ophthalmology 1987;94:1310–1314
83. Dart JK, Badenoch PR. Bacterial adherence to contact lenses. CLAO J 1986; 12:220–224
84. Fowler SA, Allansmith MR. Evaluation of soft contact lens coatings. Arch Ophthalmol 1980;98:95–99
85. Stern GA, Zam ZS. The pathogenesis of CL-associated *Pseudomonas aeruginosa* corneal ulceration. The effect of contact lens coatings on adherence of *P. aeruginosa* to SCL. Cornea 1986;5:41–45
86. Fowler SA, Greiner JV, Allansmith MR. Attachment of bacteria to soft contact lenses. Arch Ophthalmol 1979;97:659–660
87. Fowler SA, Allansmith MR. The surface of the continuously worn contact lens. Arch Ophthalmol 1980;98:1233–1236
88. Liotet S, Guillaumin D, Cochet P, et al. The genesis of organic deposits on soft contact lenses. CLAO J 1983;9:49–56
89. John T, Refojo MF, Hanninen L, et al. Adherence of viable and non-viable bacteria to soft contact lenses. Cornea 1989;8:21–33
90. Fowler SA, Allansmith MR. The effect of cleaning soft contact lenses. A scanning electron microscopic study. Arch Ophthalmol 1981;99:1382–1386
91. John T, Desai D, Sahm D. Adherence of *Acanthamoeba castellani* cysts and trophozoites to unworn soft contact lenses. Am J Ophthalmol 1989;108:658–664
92. Reichert R, Stern GA. Quantitative adherence of bacteria to human corneal epithelial cells. Arch Ophthalmol 1984;102:1394–1395
93. Stern GA, Weitzenkorn D, Valenti J. Adherence of *Pseudomonas aeruginosa* to the mouse cornea. Arch Ophthalmol 1982;100:1956–1958
94. Ramphal R, McNiece MT, Polack FP. Adherence of *Pseudomonas aeruginosa* to the injured cornea: a step in the pathogenesis of corneal infections. Ann Ophthalmol 1981;13:421–425
95. Hyndiuk RA, Davis SD, Hatchell DL, et al. Experimental *Pseudomonas* keratitis: clinical and pathological observations. Cornea 1983;2:103–114
96. Hazlett LD, Rosen D, Berk RS. Experimental eye infections caused by *Pseudomonas aeruginosa.* Ophthalmic Res 1976;8:311–317
97. Stern GA, Lubniewski A, Allen C. The interaction between *Pseudomonas aeruginosa* and the corneal epithelium. Arch Ophthalmol 1985;103:1221–1225
98. Spurr-Michaud SJ, Barza M, Gipson IK. Organ culture system for study of adher-

ence of *Pseudomonas aeruginosa* to normal and wounded corneas. Invest Ophthalmol Vis Sci 1988;29:379–386

99. DiGaetano M, Stern GA, Zam ZS. The pathogenesis of contact lens–associated *Pseudomonas aeruginosa* corneal ulceration. II: An animal model. Cornea 1986; 5:155–158

100. Duran JA, Refojo MF, Kenyon KR. Hydrogel contact lens induced *Pseudomonas* keratitis in a rabbit model. Cornea 1987;6(4):258–260

101. Koch JM, Refojo MF, Hanninen L, et al. *Pseudomonas* keratitis related to extended soft contact lens wear in a rabbit model. Invest Ophthalmol Vis Sci 1989;30(suppl):42

102. Lawin-Brussel CA, Refojo MF, Leong FL, et al. Time course of experimental *Pseudomonas aeruginosa* keratitis in contact lens overwear. Arch Ophthalmol 1990;108:1012–1019

103. Campbell J, Mehta P, Robinson D, et al. The pathogenesis of experimental *Acanthamoeba* keratitis: a morphologic study by scanning electron microscopy (SEM). Invest Ophthalmol Vis Sci 1989;30(suppl):40

104. Donzis PB, Mondino BJ, Weissman BA, et al. Microbial contamination of contact lens care systems. Am J Ophthalmol 1987;104:325–333

105. Donzis PB, Mondino BJ, Weissman BA. *Bacillus* keratitis associated with contaminated contact lens care systems. Am J Ophthalmol 1988;105:195–197

106. Donzis PB, Mondino BJ, Weissman BA, et al. Microbial analysis of contact lens care systems contaminated with *Acanthamoeba*. Am J Ophthalmol 1989;108:53–56

107. Bowden FW, Cohen EJ, Arensten JJ, et al. Patterns of lens care practices and lens product contamination in contact lens associated microbial keratitis. CLAO J 1989;15:49–54

108. Tragakis MP, Brown SL, Pearce DB. Bacteriologic studies of contamination associated with soft contact lenses. Am J Ophthalmol 1973;75:496

109. Kanpolat A, Kalayci D, Arman D, Duruk K. Contamination of contact lens care systems. CLAO J 1992;18:105–107

110. Brandt FH, Ware DH, Visvesara GS. Viability of *Acanthamoeba* cysts in ophthalmic solutions. Appl Environ Microbiol 1989;55:1144–1146

111. Ludwig IH, Meisler DM, Rutherford I, et al. Susceptibility of *Acanthamoeba* to soft contact lens disinfection systems. Invest Ophthalmol Vis Sci 1986;27:626–628

112. Wilhelmus KR. Microbial keratitis associated with contact lens wear. In: Dabezies OH Jr, ed. The CLAO guide to basic science and clinical practice, ed 2, vol 2. Boston: Little, Brown, 1988:41.1–41.18

113. Stein RM, Clinch TE, Cohen EJ, et al. Infected versus sterile corneal infiltrates in contact lens wearers. Am J Ophthalmol 1988;105:632–636

114. Liesegang TJ. Bacterial and fungal keratitis. In: Kaufman HE, McDonald MB, Barron BA, Waltman SR, eds. The cornea. New York: Churchill Livingstone, 1989:217–270

115. Belmont JB, Osler HB, Chandler RD, Schwab I. Noninfectious ring-shaped keratitis associated with *Pseudomonas aeruginosa*. Am J Ophthalmol 1982;93:338–341

116. Mondino BJ, Rabin BS, Kessler E, et al. Corneal rings with gram negative bacteria. Arch Ophthalmol 1977;95:2222–2225

117. Case records of the Massachusetts General Hospital. Weekly clinicopathological exercises (case 10). N Engl J Med 1985;312:634–641

118. Wilhelmus KR, Osato MS, Font RL, et al. Rapid diagnosis of *Acanthamoeba* keratitis using calcofluor white. Arch Ophthalmol 1986;104:1309–1312

119. Davis RM, Schroeder RP, Ramsey JJ, et al. *Acanthamoeba* keratitis and infectious crystalline keratopathy. Arch Ophthalmol 1987;105:1524–1527

120. Key SN, Green WR, Willaert E, et al. Keratitis due to *Acanthamoeba castellani*. A clinicopathologic case report. Arch Ophthalmol 1980;98:475–479

121. Moore MB. *Acanthamoeba* keratitis associated with contact lens wear. In: Dabezies

OH Jr, ed. The CLAO guide to basic science and clinical practice, ed 2, vol 2. Boston: Little, Brown, 1989:42A.1–42A.17

122. Lindquist TD, Fritsche TR, Grutzmacher RD. Scleral ectasia secondary to *Acanthamoeba* keratitis. Cornea 1990;9:74–76

123. Soloman JM, Hyndiuk RA, Koenig SB, Gradus MS. *Acanthamoeba* keratitis masquerading as corneal homograft rejection. Arch Ophthalmol 1987;105:1326–1327

124. Marines HM, Osato MS, Font RL. The value of calcofluor white in the diagnosis of mycotic and *Acanthamoeba* infections of the eye and ocular adnexa. Ophthalmology 1987;94:23–26

125. Mathers W, Stevens G, Rodrigues M, et al. Immunopathology and electron microscopy of *Acanthamoeba* keratitis. Am J Ophthalmol 1987;103:626–635

126. McClellan KA, Kappagoda NK, Filipic M, et al. Microbiological and histopathological confirmation of acanthamoebic keratitis. Pathology 1988;20:70–73

127. Robin JB, Chan R, Rao NA, et al. Fluorescein-conjugated lectin visualization of fungi and *Acanthamoeba* in infectious keratitis. Ophthalmology 1989;96:1198–1202

128. Gradus MS, Koenig SB, Hyndiuk RA, DeCarlo J. Filter-culture technique using ameoba saline transport medium for the noninvasive diagnosis of *Acanthamoeba* keratitis. Am J Ophthalmol 1989;92:682–685

129. Lindquist TD, Cameron JD, Havener VR, et al. Unsuspected infectious keratitis in host corneal buttons. Surv Ophthalmol 1989;33:359–365

130. Cokingtin CD, Hyndiuk RA. Insights from experimental data on ciprofloxacin in the treatment of bacterial keratitis and ocular infections. Am J Ophthalmol 1991;112:25S–28S

131. Wolfson JS, Hooper DC. The fluoroquinolones: structures, mechanisms of action and resistance, and spectra of activity in vitro. Antimicrob Agents Chemother 1985;28:581–586

132. Neu HC. Microbiologic aspects of fluoroquinolones. Am J Ophthalmol 1991;112:15S–24S

133. Borrmann LR, Leopold IH. The potential use of quinolones in future ocular antimicrobial therapy. Am J Ophthalmol 1988;106:227–229

134. Leibowitz HM. Clinical evaluation of ciprofloxacin 0.3% ophthalmic solution for treatment of bacterial keratitis. Am J Ophthalmol 1991;112:34S–47S

135. Mills RA, Osato MS, Pyron M, Jones DB. Efficacy of topical ceftazidime in experimental bacterial keratitis. Invest Ophthalmol Vis Sci 1992(suppl);33(4):935

136. Cutarelli PE, Lass JH, Lazarus HM, et al. Topical fluoroquinolones: antimicrobial activity and in vitro corneal epithelial toxicity. Curr Eye Res 1991;10:557–563

137. Osato MS, Jensen HG, Trousdale MD, et al. The comparative in vitro activity of ofloxacin and selected ophthalmic antimicrobial agents against ocular bacterial isolates. Am J Ophthalmol 1989;108:380–386

138. O'Brien TP, Sawusch MR, Dick SD, Gottsch JD. Topical ciprofloxacin treatment of *Pseudomonas* keratitis in rabbits. Arth Ophthalmol 1988;106:1444–1446

139. Friedberg ML, Pleyer U, Mondino BJ. Device drug delivery to the eye. Collagen shields, iontophoresis, and pumps. Ophthalmology 1991;98:725–732

140. Silbiger J, Stern GA. Evaluation of corneal collagen shields as a drug delivery device for the treatment of experimental *Pseudomonas* keratitis. Ophthalmology 1992;99:889–892

141. Sawusch MR, O'Brien TP, Dick JD, Gottsch JD. Use of collagen corneal shields in the treatment of bacterial keratitis. Am J Ophthalmol 1988;106:279–281

142. Hobden JA, Reidy JJ, O'Callaghan RJ, et al. Treatment of experimental *Pseudomonas* keratitis using collagen shields containing tobramycin. Arch Ophthalmol 1988;106:1605–1607

143. Phinney RB, Schwartz SD, Lee DA, Mondino BJ. Collagen-shield delivery of gentamicin and vancomycin. Arch Ophthalmol 1988;106:1599–1604

144. Unterman SR, Rootman DS, Hill JM, et al. Collagen shield drug delivery: thera-

peutic concentrations of tobramycin in the rabbit cornea and aqueous humor. J Cataract Refract Surg 1988;14:500–504

145. O'Brien TP, Sawusch MR, Dick JD, et al. Use of collagen corneal shields versus soft contact lenses to enhance penetration of topical tobramycin. J Cataract Refract Surg 1988;14:505–507

146. Wright P, Warhurst D, Jones BR. *Acanthamoeba* keratitis successfully treated medically. Br J Ophthalmol 1985;69:778–782

147. Berger ST, Mondino BJ, Hoft RH, et al. Successful medical management of *Acanthamoeba* keratitis. Am J Ophthalmol 1990;110:395–403

148. Ishibashi Y, Matsumoto Y, Kabata T, et al. Oral itraconazole and topical miconazole with debridement for *Acanthamoeba* keratitis. Am J Ophthalmol 1990; 109:121–126

149. Davis SD, Sarff LD, Hyndiuk RA. Corticosteroid in experimentally induced *Pseudomonas* keratitis. Arch Ophthalmol 1978;96:126–128

150. Leibowitz HM, Kupferman A. Topically administered corticosteroids. Effect of antibiotic-treated bacterial keratitis. Arch Ophthalmol 1980;98:1287–1290

151. Stern GA, Okumoto M, Friedlaender M, Smolin G. The effect of combined gentamicin-corticosteroid treatment on gentamicin-resistant *Pseudomonas* keratitis. Ann Ophthalmol 1980;12:1011–1014

152. Badenoch PR, Hay GJ, McDonald PJ, Coster DJ. A rat model of bacterial keratitis: effect of antibiotics and corticosteroids. Arch Ophthalmol 1985;103:718–720

153. Smolin G, Okumoto M, Leong-Sit L. Combined gentamicin-tobramycin-corticosteroid treatment. II. Effect on gentamicin-resistant *Pseudomonas* keratitis. Arch Ophthalmol 1980;98:473–474

154. Harbin T. Recurrence of a corneal *Pseudomonas* infection after topical steroid therapy. Am J Ophthalmol 1974;58:670–675

155. Carmichael TR, Gelfand Y, Welsh NH. Topical steroids in the treatment of central and paracentral ulcers. Br J Ophthalmol 1990;74:528–531

156. Osato MS, Robinson NM, Wilhelmus KR, Jones DB. Morphogenesis of *Acanthamoeba castellani*. Titration of the steroid effect. Invest Ophthalmol Vis Sci 1986; 27(suppl):37

157. Rabinovitch T, Weissman SS, Sheppard JD, Ostler HB. *Acanthamoeba* keratitis: clinical signs and predictions of outcome. Invest Ophthalmol Vis Sci 1989 (suppl);30:38

158. Holland GN, Donzis PB. Rapid resolution of early *Acanthamoeba* keratitis after epithelial debridement. Am J Ophthalmol 1987;104:87–89

159. Portnoy SL, Insler MS, Kaufman HE. Surgical management of corneal ulceration and perforation. Surv Ophthalmol 1989;34:47–58

160. Eiferman RA, Snyder JW. Antibacterial effect of cyanoacrylate glue. Arch Ophthalmol 1983;101:958–960

161. Hyndiuk RA, Hull DS, Kinyoun JL. Free tissue patch and cyanoacrylate in corneal perforations. Ophthalmic Surg 1974;5:50–55

162. Alpren TVP, Hyndiuk RA, Davis SD, Sarff LD. Cryotherapy for experimental *Pseudomonas* keratitis. Arch Ophthalmol 1979;97:711–714

163. Meisler DM, Ludwig FH, Rutherford I, et al. Susceptibility of *Acanthamoeba* to cryotherapeutic method. Arch Ophthalmol 1986;104:130–131

164. Binder PS. Cryotherapy for medically unresponsive *Acanthamoeba* keratitis. Cornea 1989;8:106–114

165. Freeman MI. Patient selection. Ophthalmol Clin North Am 1989;2:217–228

166. Finnemore VM. Is the dry eye contact lens wearer at risk? Not usually. Cornea 1990;9(suppl):S51–S53

167. Lemp MA. Is the dry eye contact lens wearer at risk? Yes. Cornea 1990;9(suppl): S48–S50

168. Stein HA, Slatt BJ, Stein RM. Assessment of the prospective contact lens wearer. In: Klein E, ed. Fitting guide for rigid and soft contact lenses. A practical approach. St Louis: Mosby, 1990:31–38

169. Key JE, Mobley CL. Preventing problems with current care systems. Ophthalmol Clin North Am 1989;2:339–350

170. Sibley MJ. Soft contact lens hygiene: an overview. In: Dabezies OH Jr, ed. The CLAO guide to basic and clinical practice, ed 2, vol 2. Boston: Little, Brown, 1988:40.1–40.27

171. Krezanoski JZ, Dabezies OH Jr. Hard lens hygiene. In: Dabezies OH Jr, ed. The CLAO guide to basic and clinical practice, ed 2, vol 1. Boston: Little, Brown, 1984:31.1–31.7

172. Hartstein J, Williams K. Answering patients' questions. Ophthalmol Clin North Am 1989;2:211–216

173. Preschel N, McCormick S, Shah M. A simple, effective method for sterilization of contact lens cases. Invest Ophthalmol Vis Sci 1992;33(suppl):938

174. Cohen EJ. Is your office safe? Yes. Cornea 1990;9(suppl):S41–S43

175. Centers for Disease Control. Update: universal precautions for prevention of transmission of human immunodeficiency virus, hepatitis B virus, and other bloodborne pathogens in health-care settings. MMWR 1988;37:82, 387–388

176. Centers for Disease Control. Recommendations for preventing possible transmission of human T-lymphotropic virus type III/lymphadenopathy-associated virus from tears. MMWR 1985;34:533–534

177. American Academy of Ophthalmology. Controlling risks of the possible transmission of human immunodeficiency virus (clinical alert 2/4). San Francisco: American Academy of Ophthalmology, 1988

178. Vogt MW, Ho DD, Bakar SR, et al. Safe disinfection of contact lenses after contamination with HTLV-III. Ophthalmology 1986;93:771–774

179. Lippman RE. The FDA rule in contact lens development and safety. Cornea 1990;9(suppl):S64–S68

Postoperative Endophthalmitis: Pathogenesis, Prophylaxis, and Management

Mark G. Speaker, M.D., Ph.D.

Jerry A. Menikoff, M.D.

Postoperative endophthalmitis remains one of the most devastating complications of intraocular surgery. Although acute postoperative endophthalmitis occurs relatively rarely, that fact is of little consequence to the affected patients whose experience with a vision-threatening complication is far different from their expectations of modern eye surgery. Fortunately, with recent advances in our understanding of this infection, there is increased hope of improving prophylaxis and treatment. There are a number of clinical settings in which endophthalmitis occurs, including non-infectious, endogenous, and posttraumatic circumstances, yet we limit our discussion here to cases of infectious origin that occur in the days or weeks after an intraocular operation—that is, to acute postoperative endophthalmitis.

■ Pathogenesis

To better understand the pathogenesis of postoperative endophthalmitis, we must answer a number of basic questions, such as: (1) What is the source of the infecting organisms? (2) How do they enter the eye? (3) Why do some patients but not others develop endophthalmitis?

Source of Organisms

There are occasional reports of infection having been caused by an identifiable source. Thus, there have been outbreaks of endophthalmitis due to inadequately sterilized irrigation solutions [1], contaminated intra-ocular lenses [2], and donor corneas [3]. Nonetheless, it is generally be-

"

lieved that the majority of cases are attributable to bacteria colonizing the patient, particularly the eyelid margin and conjunctiva [4, 5]. The external ocular tissues of most patients are known to be heavily colonized by organisms that are capable of causing acute postoperative endophthalmitis [6–8]. As early as 1960, Locatcher-Khorazo and Guttierrez [9] attempted to use phage typing of bacteria to elucidate the pathogenetic role of these bacteria. These techniques, however, were inadequate for demonstrating genetic identity between bacteria. Recently, we have used DNA fingerprinting to trace the origin of organisms isolated from the aqueous and vitreous of endophthalmitis patients to the patient's eyelid, conjunctiva, or nose in the majority of cases [10]. Using these highly sensitive techniques, the organisms obtained from external and intraocular sources were determined to be genetically indistinguishable in 82% of the cases examined.

These observations about the source of infecting organisms in postoperative endophthalmitis are useful in designing improved prophylactic regimens and guiding further investigation concerning the pathogenesis of such infections. However, the surgeon should not interpret these findings as evidence that standard infection control practices in the operating room are less important. The threat of infection from operating room personnel, instruments, and solutions is ever present and must be controlled vigilantly. It has been suggested that conversation between operating room personnel increases the number of airborne organisms in the surgical environment [11]. In fact, in one unusual case, we traced the source of the infecting organism to a member of the operating team who had respiratory tract disease.

Consistent with these findings, the most common organism causing postoperative endophthalmitis is also the primary bacterium colonizing the eyelid margin and conjunctiva—*Staphylococcus epidermidis* and other coagulase-negative staphylococci, organisms that, until recently, were believed to be of limited pathogenic potential [8, 12]. Coagulase-negative staphylococci are reported to cause up to 50% or more of all cases [5, 13–15] and, at our institution, they accounted for almost 90% of cases last year. In nearly a tie for a distant second place are somewhat more virulent organisms—*Staphylococcus aureus* and streptococci—together accounting for approximately 10 to 40% of cases [5, 13, 15]. Infections due to gram-negative rods such as *Pseudomonas*, *Proteus*, and *Citrobacter* species [5, 13, 16] are fortunately quite uncommon today. *Candida albicans* and other fungi are seen relatively rarely; they are most likely to be seen in circumstances favoring opportunistic infections, such as in immunosuppressed patients [17]. The prognosis for recovery of useful vision after infection with the more virulent organisms such as *S. aureus*, streptococci, and particularly the gram-negative rods, is less favorable, as discussed in more detail later.

The current prevalence of *S. epidermidis* in postoperative endophthalmitis raises unresolved questions concerning whether the pathogenic origin of endophthalmitis has changed over time. As recently as the early

1970s, most studies suggested that the majority of cases were due to relatively virulent bacteria, with approximately 50% caused by *S. aureus* and another 25% by gram-negative rods [18]. It is possible that this apparent shift in pathogens is due in part to the failure to recognize *S. epidermidis* as an intraocular pathogen, which was first demonstrated by Valenton and colleagues in 1973 [19, 20]. It is unlikely to be due to changes in ocular flora [8] but rather to changes in surgical technique, such as the insertion of intraocular lenses (IOLs), which provide a binding site for relatively nonvirulent organisms, as well as increased instrumentation and irrigation [13]. The recognition of *S. epidermidis* as a significant pathogen elsewhere in the body, especially in connection with blood infections, appears to be similarly related to the increased use of prosthetic intravascular devices [21].

Special forms of endophthalmitis are associated with distinctive groups of pathogens. For example, bleb-related endophthalmitis is usually caused by more virulent organisms such as *S. aureus,* streptococcal species, and *Hemophilus influenzae* [22], whereas many cases of chronic endophthalmitis are caused by less virulent anaerobic organisms such as *Propionibacterium acnes* [23].

Routes of Bacterial Entry

It is assumed that the infecting organisms are usually introduced into the eye through incision sites at the time of intraocular surgery [17]. During cataract extraction, for example, samples of aqueous fluid have been culture-positive in up to 43% of cases [24, 25]. Irrigation fluids and surgical instruments can play a role in carrying into the eye bacteria that colonize the eyelid or conjunctiva, as can IOLs. IOLs placed directly on the external ocular surface at the beginning of an operation were demonstrated to be culture-positive in 26% of cases [26]. Electrostatic forces may allow bacteria to adhere to the lens surface as it passes across the eyelid margin or through the external aspect of the wound [27].

Introduction of organisms into the eye postoperatively can also lead to endophthalmitis. Vitreous wicks [28] and inadequately buried sutures [29] can provide a route for bacterial entry. Relatively innocuous procedures such as removal of sutures [30] can lead to endophthalmitis, as can procedures that are ordinarily not intraocular, such as strabismus surgery [31] or radial keratotomy [32]. In the latter instances, it appears that inadvertent penetration of the globe usually has occurred. Driebe and colleagues [33], in a survey of 83 cases, reported that in 22% of these cases, wound abnormalities were noted at the time that endophthalmitis was diagnosed. We have not observed wound abnormalities in eyes with endophthalmitis with the same frequency as Driebe and colleagues, and the relationship of these abnormalities to the pathogenesis of endophthalmitis is unclear. It has been suggested that sutureless cataract extraction procedures may allow postoperative entry of bacteria into the eye, leading to endophthalmitis [34]. This seems likely, however, only if the incision is not truly self-sealing. Endophthalmitis occurring months or years after a glaucoma filtering procedure is believed to occur owing to entry of bacteria through the filtering bleb [22, 35]. Of great interest are reports regarding the development of acute endophthalmitis after laser capsulotomy [36], where the procedure appears to allow organisms of low virulence, such as *S. epidermidis* or *P. acnes,* to be released into the vitreous from their occult sequestration within the capsular bag.

Risk Factors

Although there are several sources of evidence to suggest that entry of bacteria into the eye at the time of operation is common, a relatively small percentage of patients develop endophthalmitis. Recent reports of the incidence of postoperative endophthalmitis range from approximately 0.1 to 0.4% [5, 16, 37, 38]. This compares very favorably to the rate of infection after surgical procedures on other parts of the body, which is approximately 3% for clean wounds [39]. Nationwide statistics from the Medicare database analyzed by Javitt and associates [37] give rates of 0.085% for extracapsular extraction and phacoemulsification and 0.11% for intracapsular extraction. All these rates are significantly reduced from those reported decades earlier, which were as high as 0.7% [5]. One reason for this change may be that improved surgical techniques and antimicrobials led to a reduction in the number of bacteria inoculated into the eye intraoperatively [25].

Although the anterior chamber appears to be relatively efficient at clearing small numbers of bacteria [40], we do not understand the reasons for the failure of this mechanism in some patients. In an individual case of endophthalmitis due to coagulase-negative staphylococci, we have not yet been able to determine whether the occurrence of infection is related to the size of the bacterial inoculum, the virulence of the infecting strain of *Staphylococcus,* deficits in local host defenses that are either preexisting or induced by the operation, or systemic deficits in host immunity related to disease such as diabetes mellitus. It is likely to be the case that an individual patient's risk of developing endophthalmitis is multifactorial, and better identification of risk factors for endophthalmitis is therefore important.

Vitreous Communication   The vitreous appears to play a major role in the development of endophthalmitis. In contrast to the anterior chamber, elimination of bacteria from the vitreous cavity appears to be much less efficient; however, the reason for this is unknown. Perhaps it can be explained by the difficulty in moving cells and soluble immune mediators through the viscous vitreous gel or by unique properties of the vitreous as a culture medium [41]. Several studies have demonstrated a higher incidence of endophthalmitis in cases where bacteria have access to the vitreous, such as through a posterior capsular tear [33, 37, 38, 41]. This may, in part, explain the higher rate of endophthalmitis for intracapsular, as opposed to extracapsular, cataract extraction [37]. In a recent case-control study of postoperative endophthalmitis performed at our institution, we determined that such communication with the vitreous cavity—defined to include procedures in which there was either a defect in the posterior lens capsule or zonules or vitreous instrumentation was part of the procedure—can increase the risk of endophthalmitis by a factor of nearly 14 [38].

Intraocular Lenses A number of recent studies indicate that IOLs generally, and particularly those made with certain materials, may be risk factors for the development of endophthalmitis. These plastic prosthetic devices can act as sites for the binding of bacteria, which can then shelter themselves from the patient's immune system by secreting protective slimes [23, 27, 42, 43]. Dilly and Holmes Sellors [44] observed that bacteria appear to bind better to polypropylene (Prolene) than to polymethylmethacrylate (PMMA). Our recent epidemiological study suggests that the use of IOLs with Prolene haptics increases the risk of endophthalmitis by a factor of 4.5 [38]. Using quantitative laboratory techniques, we have recently confirmed that coagulase-negative staphylococci preferentially adhere to IOLs with Prolene haptics compared to all-PMMA lenses [45]. Although many surgeons have used IOLs with Prolene haptics for many years without incident, our epidemiological data suggest that the total number of cases of endophthalmitis occurring annually in the United States could be reduced from 1,200 to 500 by avoiding such IOLs, thus saving 700 patients each year from a potentially devastating complication.

Diabetes and Other Patient Characteristics Specific deficits in the immune system may also play a role in the development of endophthalmitis. Thus, patients who are immunosuppressed or who have the acquired immunodeficiency syndrome (AIDS) may be particularly susceptible, and the case reports largely relate to endogenous infection, with the bacteria or fungi reaching the eye by way of the bloodstream [17]. With regard to postoperative endophthalmitis, however, there is clinical evidence that diabetics are particularly at risk [5, 13, 16]. This finding is consistent with the observation that diabetics have impaired resistance to other infections [46].

■ Diagnosis

A critical element in the successful treatment of postoperative endophthalmitis is early diagnosis and prompt intervention. Early diagnosis requires maintaining a high index of suspicion in surgical patients with intraocular inflammation that is more severe than expected [47]. Some of the most common findings—pain, conjunctival injection, and eyelid edema [48]—are not completely reliable, as patients with infections due, to low-virulence organisms may present without pain or extraordinary external inflammation. Loss of vision due to the formation of an inflammatory pupillary membrane, opacification of the vitreous with diminution of the red reflex, or hypopyon (Fig 1) are more consistent findings associated with acute postoperative infection. Accordingly, patients should be instructed concerning the expected postoperative course and the need to seek help immediately if they experience pain or loss of vision. Special risk factors, such as whether the procedure was long and complicated, whether the patient was a diabetic, or whether there was a defect in the intact posterior capsule, should also be kept in mind, and some patients should be followed more closely than others. If uncertainty exists concerning a case of suspected endophthalmitis, the patient should be carefully observed over a period of hours while he or she refrains from eating or drinking, so that surgical intervention is not delayed in the event that it is required. It is not advisable to send these patients home to return for examination the next day if significant doubt exists, since the infection can progress very rapidly.

In general, more virulent organisms will produce the earliest onset of symptoms and the most dramatic presentation. Thus, a case that is clinically obvious within 1 to 3 postoperative days is most likely to be caused by *S. aureus*, streptococci, or gram-negative rods. In contrast, patients who develop symptoms a week or more postoperatively are more likely to be infected with organisms such as *S. epidermidis* [20, 49]. These are merely generalizations, however, and the time of presentation can be highly variable. Fungi will not present until 3 to 4 weeks after the procedure and will produce fluffy white exudates, like puff-balls, in the vitreous [4]. Truly slow-acting bacteria, such as *P. acnes,* usually will produce only subtle signs and symptoms and often not until months have passed [23].

Intraocular Cultures

When a patient presents with signs and symptoms that are suggestive of infectious endophthalmitis, the accepted approach is to obtain intraocu-

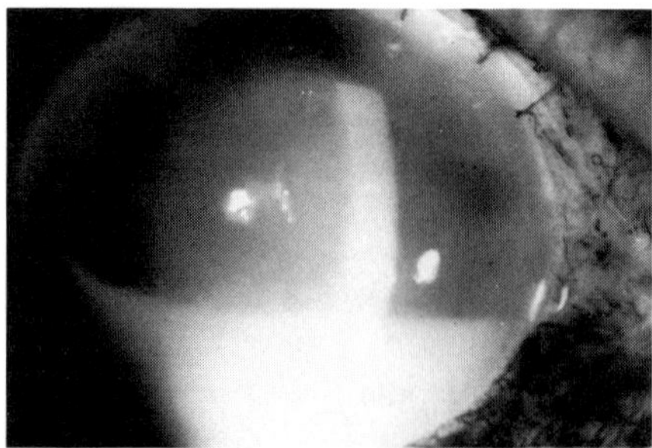

Figure 1 *Staphylococcal endophthalmitis presenting 3 days after cataract extraction, with the typical appearance of corneal edema and hypopyon.*

lar samples for culture. External cultures of the eyelid margins, conjunctiva, and nasal cavity often will yield the same organism that is growing inside the eye [10]. However, it is impossible to differentiate the true infecting organism from other species of bacteria that may be colonizing the patient's external tissues, except by molecular genetics [10, 50]. We routinely recommend that external cultures be obtained, since demonstration of the infecting organism as part of the patient's normal flora may be of some use to the surgeon in explaining the pathogenesis of the infection to the patient or, alternatively, in a medicolegal setting. Whenever possible, samples should be taken from both the aqueous and the vitreous, prior to institution of intensive topical, systemic, or intraocular antibiotic therapy. Obtaining a vitreous sample is by far the most important, since aqueous samples have been demonstrated to be negative in up to 57% of cases in which culture-positive vitreous samples were obtained [20].

Vitreous specimens for culture should be obtained with an automated vitreous cutting instrument using trans–pars plana technique. Aspiration of fluid from the vitreous cavity using a syringe usually is difficult and probably places undesirable traction on an inflamed and friable retina. The pars plana sclerotomy sites should be prepared prior to obtaining a sample of aqueous through a limbal stab incision. A pupillary membrane is invariably present that can be removed with a forceps or cystotome needle after filling the anterior chamber with a viscoelastic substance. Removal of the pupillary membrane is essential to obtaining adequate visualization of the vitreous cavity for the vitrectomy.

The vitrectomy instrument should be prepared with a tubing set that allows insertion of a three-way stopcock and a 10-ml collection syringe in the aspiration line. The initial 1-ml vitrectomy specimen should be collected via the stopcock with the syringe, prior to turning on the infusion port, which allows the most concentrated material to be collected for culture. This undiluted vitreous is the most important material for culture, and both the aqueous and vitreous specimens should be separately dripped without delay onto the center of agar plates that have equilibrated to room temperature. The remainder of the vitrectomy fluid can be collected from the cassette, and the relatively dilute fluid can be centrifuged to produce a concentrated pellet. This pellet can be stained and examined under the microscope or cultured after resuspension in a small volume of sterile saline. Alternatively, the fluid from the cassette can be cultured by running it through a 0.45-μm filter to concentrate it, with cut-up pieces of the filter paper being directly placed on the agar plates [51]. Appropriate culture media for bacteria include blood agar (aerobic and anaerobic), chocolate agar, and thioglycolate broth, all incubated at 37°C. In addition, room-temperature cultures on Sabouraud's agar are needed to grow fungi. Slides of the specimens should also be examined for organisms after Gram and Giemsa staining. We usually keep a portion of the concentrated vitrectomy specimen for electron microscopy. A positive culture result is commonly defined as growth of the same organism on two different media, confluent growth on a solid medium, or any anaerobic growth in the anaerobic media [52].

Negative cultures from aqueous and vitreous were obtained in 30% of the last 100 cases at our institution. Negative cultures do not usually preclude the presence of infection but probably reflect sterilization of the infection by host defenses [53], sequestration of organisms within phagocytes, infection by fastidious organisms, or poor technique in handling of the cultures. Electron microscopy has been helpful in demonstrating microorganisms within phagocytes in cases where cultures have remained negative. It has been demonstrated by Pokorny and colleagues [54] that sonication of vitreous specimens prior to culture can release organisms that are trapped within phagocytes and convert specimens from culture-negative to culture-positive.

Differential Diagnosis

The differential diagnosis of acute postoperative endophthalmitis should include sterile uveitis (due to retained lens material or foreign materials introduced during operation), sympathetic ophthalmia, preexisting uveitis, or iris trauma. Sterile uveitis, which has been reported to occur in as many as 2% of patients following cataract extraction, rarely will cause pain or severe visual deterioration, although occasionally it may produce a hypopyon [4]. Nonetheless, if there is the slightest suspicion of bacterial endophthalmitis, we believe it is best to err on the side of caution and proceed with cultures and treatment as if the patient does have a bacterial infection. Even with the least virulent species of bacteria, which are most likely to produce milder presenting symptoms, significant visual loss can occur if treatment is delayed [5, 15].

■ Treatment

One of the most important aspects of the treatment of postoperative endophthalmitis is early diagnosis and prompt institution of effective antimicrobial therapy. It is important that operating room personnel and other surgeons understand the emergent nature of endophthalmitis, as operating room schedules often must be interrupted to accommodate these cases. At our institution, a policy has been established that specifically addresses the priority nature of endophthalmitis cases.

As discussed earlier, the spectrum of pathogens depends on the clinical setting in which endophthalmitis occurs. The comments herein concern treatment of acute postoperative endophthalmitis. Even though the predominant pathogens today are coagulase-negative staphylococci, broad-spectrum antimicrobial therapy must be instituted initially to cover the full range of potential bacterial pathogens including streptococci and gram-negative rods. Current therapy consists of intravitreal, systemic, and topical antibiotics, usually combined with vitrectomy (Table 1). The role of systemic antibiotics and vitrectomy in the treatment of endophthalmitis has been somewhat controversial, and a study sponsored by the National Institutes of Health, the Endophthalmitis Vitrectomy Study (EVS), is currently being conducted to address these issues.

Intravitreal and Topical Antibiotics

For more than a decade, there has been agreement that direct intravitreal injection of antibiotics is a mainstay of treatment [55], allowing effective intraocular concentrations of antibiotics to be achieved immediately after injection. Previous attempts to treat with only intravenous, topical, and subconjunctival antibiotics produced inconsistent results, presumably due to poor antibiotic penetration into the vitreous. Experimental evidence suggests that significant penetration of antibiotics administered intravenously may take as long as 48 hours. The choice of intravitreal drugs for acute postoperative endophthalmitis represents a broad consensus and

Table 1 *Recommendations for Treatment of Acute Postoperative Endophthalmitis*

Swab cultures of eyelid margins and conjunctiva of both eyes and nasal mucosa

Diagnostic vitrectomy and anterior chamber paracentesis for culture and sensitivity
    Aerobic and anaerobic blood agar
    Chocolate agar
    Sabouraud's agar
    Thioglycolate broth
    Gram stain
    Electron microscopy

Therapeutic vitrectomy (optional)

Intravitreal antibiotics
    Ceftazidime, 2.25 mg in 0.1 ml water, *or*
    Amikacin, 400 µg in 0.1 ml water, *and*
    Vancomycin, 1,000 µg in 0.1 ml water

Intravitreal corticosteroid
    Dexamethasone, 360 µg in 0.1 ml water

Intravenous antibiotics (dosage must be adjusted according to patient's weight and renal function)
    Vancomycin, 1 gm every 12 hours (infusion rate ≤ 10 mg/min)
    Ceftazidime, 2 gm every 8 hours

Intravenous corticosteroids (when not contraindicated)
    Methylprednisolone sodium succinate (Solu-Medrol), 40–80 mg/day for 3–5 days

Topical antibiotics
    Gentamicin, 14 mg/ml, and vancomycin, 25 mg/ml
                or
    Ciprofloxacin 0.3%

consists of an aminoglycoside with a broad spectrum of activity against gram-negative bacilli and staphylococci, combined with vancomycin (1,000 μg), which extends the coverage against gram-positive organisms, particularly streptococci and methicillin-resistant staphylococci. Concern over the numerous case reports of retinal toxicity from aminoglycosides [56], especially when used in combination with vancomycin, has led to a shift away from the use of gentamicin (100 μg) in preference of amikacin (400 μg), which is believed to be less toxic [57]. Ceftazidime (2.25 mg), a third-generation cephalosporin with excellent activity against pseudomonas and staphylococci and less toxicity than aminoglycosides, can be used in place of amikacin. Each of these antibiotics should be injected slowly in a 0.1-ml volume into the anterior vitreous, with the bevel of a 22-gauge needle facing anteriorly [48]. The need for vancomycin has come about because of the increased incidence of methicillin (oxacillin) resistance among staphylococcal isolates from endophthalmitis cases [58], which at our institution is approximately 40%. In the EVS, all patients will receive intravitreal injections of amikacin (0.4 mg) and vancomycin (1.0 mg), with the addition of subconjunctival injections of vancomycin (25 mg) and ceftazidime (100 mg) [59].

Although repeat intravitreal injection of antibiotics 48 to 96 hours after the initial injection has been proposed as possibly beneficial, we avoid repeat injections because of the risk of increased retinal toxicity. All EVS patients will also receive topical vancomycin and amikacin and topical cycloplegics, although the efficacy of such treatment is largely undemonstrated. Subconjunctival antibiotics are rarely used to treat endophthalmitis [52].

Corticosteroids

We routinely use intravitreal dexamethasone (360 μg), administered in conjunction with the intravitreal antibiotics, in all cases of acute postoperative endophthalmitis unless fungal infection is suspected. In addition, we give intravenous methylprednisolone sodium succinate (Solu-Medrol), 40 to 80 mg/day for the first 3 to 5 days, to all patients in whom it is not contraindicated. All EVS patients will receive topical, periocular, and systemic steroids. The role of these agents remains uncertain, although one would expect exuberant inflammation in the vitreous cavity on antibiotic-mediated death of bacteria that would be ameliorated by steroids, and animal studies suggest that steroid use may improve the outcome [60].

Therapeutic Vitrectomy

A major treatment controversy concerns when, if ever, a therapeutic vitrectomy should be performed. Therapeutic pars plana vitrectomy, which is more extensive than the limited diagnostic vitrectomy performed solely for the purpose of obtaining an adequate culture, offers the advantages of removing the byproducts of inflammation and necrotic material proximal to the retina (so-called "abscess drainage") as well as allowing better circulation of antibiotics and visualization of the fundus. A common approach, which we follow, has been to distinguish between mild and severe clinical presentations. A case is usually considered severe based on a combination of profound visual loss (to hand movements or light perception) and an inability to visualize the fundus because of opacification of the vitreous [48, 51] or continued deterioration despite initial therapy [49]. Indicative of the current uncertainty is the EVS approach, which randomizes all patients between an initial pars plana vitrectomy or just a vitreous tap (for culture purposes), irrespective of the severity of the clinical presentation [59]. This approach was taken by the EVS owing to concern that the poor results reported in the literature for patients treated with vitrectomy might have been attributable to the fact that only the most severe cases were so treated.

Our approach is to perform a limited diagnostic vitrectomy and inject intravitreal antibiotics in those cases in which the fundus reflex is still present. However, these cases are the exception. In the more typical severely affected patient, with densely opacified and inflamed vitreous, a more extensive vitrectomy is performed. The posterior hyaloid face often is not detached, making total vitrectomy somewhat hazardous in the presence of an inflamed retina; therefore, we are careful to avoid placing any stress on the retina. Because of the difficulty of controlling the dose of antibiotic delivered to the retina, and the demonstrated efficacy of intravitreal injection, we avoid putting antibiotics in the vitrectomy infusion fluids.

Intravenous Antibiotics

Another controversy to be addressed by the EVS is whether intravenous antibiotics are an appropriate aspect of therapy. In general, this mode of administration produces poor penetration into the vitreous of uninflamed eyes while imposing a risk of side effects. The penetration of intravenous antibiotics into the vitreous of inflamed eyes appears to be better, but it is not clear that the levels achieved are adequate to be effective. Nonetheless, we and most others continue to use intravenous antibiotics as adjunctive therapy to intravitreal antibiotics. The EVS will randomize patients to either no intravenous antibiotics or a combination of intravenous ceftazidime and amikacin. We currently favor ceftazidime and vancomycin as initial intravenous therapy, with withdrawal of vancomycin and substitution of a less toxic antibiotic once identification of the organism and sensitivities are available. Concomitant use of vancomycin with an aminoglycoside should be avoided because of potential toxicity. Once again, we use vancomycin initially because of the prevalence of methicillin resistance among the staphylococci in our area, and ceftazidime because it provides good gram-negative coverage including pseudomonads, with less risk of toxicity than the aminoglycosides. Vancomycin must be administered by slow infusion (10 mg/min or less) to avoid the "red-neck" syndrome, and the dosage of vancomycin and ceftazidime must be adjusted in the presence of impaired renal function because both are primarily excreted by the kidneys. If treatment with vancomycin is continued, then it is advisable to monitor serum concentrations. Oral ciprofloxacin is an attractive therapeutic agent because it has a broad spectrum of activity, including some methicillin-resistant staphylococci and most pseudomonads, as well as good vitreous penetration, and treatment can conveniently be continued for several days after the patient is discharged from the hospital.

Presence of an IOL

It usually is possible to sterilize the interior of the eye without removing the IOL [33], and therefore our practice is always to leave it in place. Moreover, when treating phakic patients, it may similarly be possible to preserve an uninvolved crystalline lens [61].

■ Prognosis

The visual prognosis after optimal treatment can be very good, depending in large part on the virulence of the infecting organism. Approximately one-third of patients in recent studies have achieved visual acuities of 20/60 or better [5, 15]. The best results tend to occur in patients who either were culture-negative (thus raising an issue regarding certainty of diagnosis) or had less virulent organisms, such as *S. epidermidis* [16, 62]. This is by no means a uniform finding, since severe loss of vision can ensue after appropriate treatment even when the organism is less virulent. In particular, the development of endophthalmitis after vitrectomy in a diabetic usually results in a poor outcome, even if the infecting organism is *S. epidermidis* [13, 15]. Infections with gram-negative bacteria and streptococci are usually quite fulminant, with a very poor prognosis.

■ Prevention

Preventive measures can be separated into two categories: those applied to all patients and special measures for patients at higher risk for developing intraocular infection. We encourage the routine use of plastic adhesive drapes to cover the eyelid margins and lashes so that they are effectively isolated from the operative field. In addition, we recommend

Table 2 *Recommendations for Prophylaxis of Postoperative Endophthalmitis*

Recognition and treatment of preoperative external disease

Topical antibiotics
  Ciprofloxacin 0.3% every 3 hours on the day before surgery and every 15 minutes
    × 4 prior to surgery

Topical antiseptic preparation of the eye for surgery
  Povidone-iodine 5% solution, 2 drops in the conjunctival sac
  Povidone-iodine 5% solution to the eyelid margins and lashes
  Povidone-iodine 10% solution to prepare the skin
  Saline irrigation

Adhesive-backed plastic incise drapes (e.g., #1035, 3M, St. Paul, MN) to cover the eyelid margins and lashes

Subconjunctival antibiotics or collagen shield delivery of antibiotic
  Gentamicin, 20 mg, or ceftazidime, 100 mg
                    and
  Vancomycin, 25 mg

---

the use of preoperative and perioperative topical antibiotics, preparation of the conjunctiva and eyelid margins with povidone-iodine, and subconjunctival injection of antibiotics at the end of surgery (Table 2). The efficacy of subconjunctival antibiotics is unclear, and care must be taken to avoid intraocular injection. Subconjunctival injection of aminoglycosides has been associated with severe toxic reactions [56]. In addition, our epidemiological study suggests that we should use all-PMMA IOLs and avoid lenses with Prolene haptics when possible because of the increased affinity of some bacteria for Prolene. There are varying amounts of evidence supporting the efficacy of each of these measures. Nonetheless, the need for a thorough approach to prophylaxis is compelling [63, 64], especially given the increasing evidence that the patient's own bacterial flora are transported into the eye in a high percentage of routine cataract extractions.

Topical Povidone-Iodine

The use of topical antiseptic agents for preoperative prophylaxis predates the use of topical antibiotics. Traditionally, the agent most commonly used was a silver protein solution (Argyrol). Isenberg and colleagues [65] demonstrated that this solution is virtually useless in reducing the ocular bacterial flora. In contrast, following up on the earlier work of Hale [66], these investigators showed a significant antibacterial effect from the use of 5% povidone-iodine [67].

To evaluate the efficacy of preoperative antimicrobial prophylaxis with povidone-iodine, we performed a controlled, nonrandomized study involving 8,083 patients at our institution [15]. Our results demonstrated a statistically significant reduction in the incidence of culture-positive endophthalmitis in patients treated with povidone-iodine. No adverse effects from the use of povidone-iodine have been reported in more than 20,000 patients. These results suggest that preoperative antimicrobial prophylaxis is indeed effective.

Accordingly, we now apply povidone-iodine in all intraocular surgery cases, unless the surgery involves an "open" eye (e.g., an open traumatic wound or fistula) or the patient has a known allergy to iodine. Our protocol involves using 2 drops of a 5% povidone-iodine solution, which are instilled in the conjunctival sac. This is followed by gentle manipulation of the eyelids to distribute the solution over the ocular surface. The eyelashes and eyelid margins are also scrubbed with povidone-iodine-soaked cotton swabs. The solution remains in the eye for the several minutes it takes subsequently to prepare the skin, and it is then irrigated out with saline solution. It is important to distinguish between povidone-iodine solution and povidone-iodine scrub, since the latter contains a detergent that is toxic to the eye and should never be used to prepare the conjunctival sac or eyelid margins.

The most significant reductions in periocular bacterial flora in the studies of Apt and Isenberg [65, 67] were produced by a combination of a 3-day preoperative course of topical Neosporin (polymyxin B sulfate, neomycin sulfate, and gramicidin) and 5% povidone-iodine applied as part of the preoperative preparation in the operating room.

Topical Preoperative Antibiotics

If most cases of postoperative endophthalmitis are caused by organisms colonizing the eyelid margin and conjunctiva, it would seem important to attempt to sterilize the ocular surface preoperatively. A number of studies have claimed that topical preoperative antibiotics can reduce the incidence of endophthalmitis. Most of these were not controlled studies, however, and merely compared their results to those reported elsewhere. As noted by Starr in a comprehensive review [68], the preponderance of the evidence does suggest that preoperative topical antibiotics can reduce the

---

Figure 2 *An important prophylactic measure is the application of an adehesive-backed plastic drape to cover the eyelid margins and lashes. The drape isolates this important source of staphylococci and other bacteria from the incision and prevents the instruments and intraocular lens from contacting the eyelid margin prior to entering the eye. (A) The eyelid margins are retracted with the wooden end of cotton-tipped applicator sticks, with the lashes everted and skin exposed adjacent to the lid margin to which the drape can adhere. The drape is applied first to the medial canthal area. (B) The drape is then incised exactly halfway between the eyelid margins from medial to lateral canthal areas, with additional relaxing incisions extended beyond the canthi. In addition, four incisions in the drape are placed perpendicular to the cut edge almost to the lid margin, two on the upper and two on the lower edge on each side of the corneal limbus to form an H pattern. (C) The eyelid speculum is then inserted so that the cut edges of the drape wrap around the lid margins. The speculum is inserted without otherwise retracting the eyelids, so that the lashes do not slip out from under the drape.*

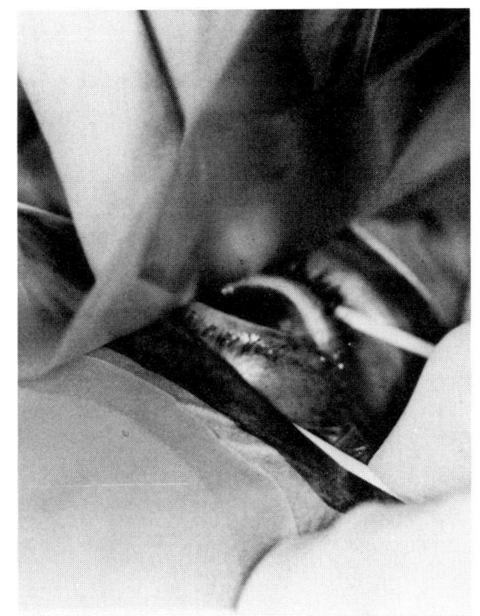

A

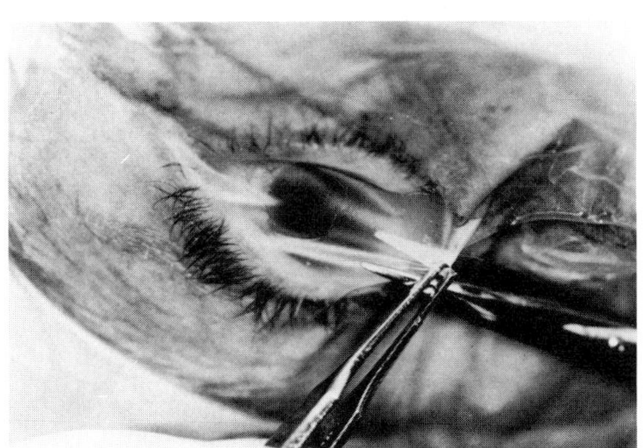

B

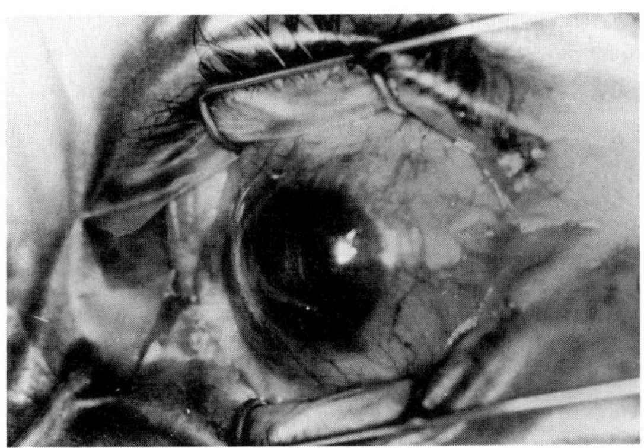

C

incidence of infection. Unfortunately, there is less guidance regarding the choice of antibiotic and the dosage, frequency, and timing of administration.

Studies of antibiotic prophylaxis in nonophthalmic surgery have demonstrated that the most effective time for administration of the antibiotics is in the 2-hour period immediately before surgery, not earlier and not postoperatively [69]. Eradication of bacteria from the eyelid margin and conjunctiva with topical antibiotics, on the other hand, is probably most effective when begun the day before operation and continued up to the time of operation. The best choice of antibiotic at this time may be a topical quinolone, such as ciprofloxacin, because it is effective against many of the methicillin-resistant staphylococci that we encounter, in contrast to the aminoglycosides. We must be concerned about the possible emergence of resistance with routine prophylactic use of any agent; however, this is less likely with a 24-hour course of treatment.

Subconjunctival Antibiotics

Subconjunctival injection of antibiotics at the end of an operation is also common, and an aminoglycoside is a frequent choice. However, experimental data show that vitreous penetration is poor, and the risk of macular infarction from subconjunctival injection of aminoglycosides is present, prompting Campochiaro and Conway [56] to recommend the abandonment of postoperative subconjunctival antibiotics. Animal studies, in contrast, do demonstrate a benefit to the addition of subconjunctival antibiotics [70]. As Meredith [64] has commented, despite the common use of this prophylactic technique, whether it really should be employed remains unclear.

Draping

As discussed earlier, adhesive-backed plastic drapes (e.g., #1035, 3M, St. Paul, MN) should be used routinely to cover the eyelids and lashes, isolating the richest source of staphylococci from the operative field. The technique is illustrated in Figure 2.

High-Risk Patients

Patients with special conditions likely to increase the ocular flora, such as chronic blepharitis or lacrimal drainage system abnormalities, should be cultured before surgery and receive appropriate topical antibiotics [48]. An unresolved question is the possible need for special prophylaxis in cases where there are risk factors for endophthalmitis, such as in a patient who is a diabetic [46] or in whom the operation is lengthy and involves much instrumentation and contact with the vitreous. Possible approaches to such patients include adding intravitreal injection of antibiotics or postoperative treatment with intensive topical or systemic antibiotics to the surgical plan.

Obviously, these approaches require the surgeon to weigh benefits versus risks of retinal and systemic toxicity without adequate information to evaluate easily either side of the equation. It is possible that a short course of an orally administered antibiotic such as ciprofloxacin, which penetrates the vitreous fairly well, would be beneficial in patients after vitreous surgery or manipulation. At the very least, however, such patients should be closely monitored during the first postoperative week.

■ References

1. Stern WH, Tamura E, Jacobs RA, et al. Epidemic postsurgical *Candida parapsilosis* endophthalmitis; clinical findings and management of 15 consecutive cases. Ophthalmology 1985;92:1701–1709
2. Gerding DN, Poley BJ, Hall WH, et al. Treatment of *Pseudomonas* endophthalmitis associated with prosthetic intraocular lens implantation. Am J Ophthalmol 1979; 88:902–908
3. Cameron JA, Antonios SR, Cotter JB, et al. Endophthalmitis from contaminated donor corneas following penetrating keratoplasty. Arch Ophthalmol 1991;109: 54–59
4. Weber DJ, Hoffman KL, Thoft RA, Baker AS. Endophthalmitis following intraocular lens implantation: report of 30 cases and review of the literature. Rev Infect Dis 1986;8:12–20
5. Kattan HM, Flynn HW Jr, Pflugfelder SC, et al. Nosocomial endophthalmitis survey: current incidence of infection after intraocular surgery. Ophthalmology 1991; 98:227–238
6. Dunnington JH, Locatcher-Khorazo D. Value of cultures before operation for cataract. Arch Ophthalmol 1945;34:215–219
7. Allansmith MR, Anderson RP, Butterworth M. The meaning of preoperative cultures in ophthalmology. Trans Am Acad Ophthalmol Otolaryngol 1969;73: 683–690
8. Walker CB, Claoue CMP. Incidence of conjunctival colonization by bacteria capable of causing postoperative endophthalmitis. J R Soc Med 1986;79:520–521
9. Locatcher-Khorazo D, Gutierrez E. Bacteriophage typing of *Staphylococcus aureus.* A study of normal, infected eyes and environment. Arch Ophthalmol 1960;63: 774–787
10. Speaker MG, Milch FA, Shah MK, et al. Role of external bacterial flora in the pathogenesis of acute postoperative endophthalmitis. Ophthalmology 1991;98: 639–650
11. Schiff FS. The shouting surgeon as a possible source of endophthalmitis. Ophthalmic Surg 1990;21:438–440
12. Perkins RE, Kundsin RB, Pratt MV, et al. Bacteriology of normal and infected conjunctiva. J Clin Microbiol 1975;1:147–149
13. Verbraeken H, Rysselaere M. Bacteriological study of 92 cases of proven infectious endophthalmitis treated with pars plana vitrectomy. Ophthalmologica 1991;203: 17–23
14. Puliafito CA, Baker AS, Haaf J, Foster CS. Infectious endophthalmitis: review of 36 cases. Ophthalmology 1982;89:921–929
15. Speaker MG, Menikoff JA. Prophylaxis of endophthalmitis with topical povidone-iodine. Ophthalmology 1991;98:1769–1775
16. Fisch A, Salvanet A, Prazuck T, et al. Epidemiology of infective endophthalmitis in France. Lancet 1991;338:1373–1376
17. Wilson FM II. Causes and prevention of endophthalmitis. Int Ophthalmol Clin 1987;27:67–73

18. Forster RK. Etiology and diagnosis of bacterial postoperative endophthalmitis. Ophthalmology 1978;85:320–326
19. Valenton MJ, Brubaker RF, Allen HF. *Staphylococcus epidermidis* (albus) endophthalmitis; report of two cases after cataract extraction. Arch Ophthalmol 1973;89:94–96
20. Bode DD Jr, Gelender H, Forster RK. A retrospective review of endophthalmitis due to coagulase-negative staphylococci. Br J Ophthalmol 1985;69:915–919
21. Schaberg DR. Major trends in the microbial etiology of nosocomial infection. Am J Med 1991;91(suppl 3B):72S–75S
22. Mandelbaum S, Forster RK, Gelender H, Culbertson W. Late onset endophthalmitis associated with filtering blebs. Ophthalmology 1985;92:964–972
23. Meisler DM, Palestine AG, Vastine DW, et al. Chronic *Propionibacterium* endophthalmitis after extracapsular cataract extraction and intraocular lens implantation. Am J Ophthalmol 1986;102:733–739
24. Sherwood DR, Rich WJ, Jacob SJ, et al. Bacterial contamination of intraocular and extraocular fluids during cataract extraction. Eye 1989;3:308–312
25. Dickey JB, Thompson KD, Jay WM. Anterior chamber aspirate cultures after uncomplicated cataract surgery. Am J Ophthalmol 1991;112:278–282
26. Vafidis GC, March RJ, Stacey AR. Bacterial contamination of intraocular lens surgery. Br J Ophthalmol 1984;68:520–523
27. Griffiths PG, Elliot TSJ, McTaggart L. Adherence of *Staphylococcus epidermidis* to intraocular lenses. Br J Ophthalmol 1989;73:402–406
28. Lindstrom RL, Doughman DJ. Bacterial endophthalmitis associated with vitreous wick. Ann Ophthalmol 1979;11:1775–1778
29. Confino J, Brown SI. Bacterial endophthalmitis associated with exposed monofilament sutures following corneal transplantation. Am J Ophthalmol 1985;99:111–113
30. Gelender H. Bacterial endophthalmitis following cutting of sutures after cataract surgery. Am J Ophthalmol 1982;94:528–533
31. Salamon SM, Friberg TR, Luxenberg MN. Endophthalmitis after strabismus surgery. Am J Ophthalmol 1982;93:39–41
32. Gelender H, Flynn HW Jr, Mandelbaum SH. Bacterial endophthalmitis resulting from radial keratotomy. Am J Ophthalmol 1982;93:323–326
33. Driebe WT Jr, Mandelbaum S, Forster RK, et al. Pseudophakic endophthalmitis: diagnosis and management. Ophthalmology 1986;93:442–448
34. Stonecipher KG, Parmley VC, Jensen H, Rowsey JJ. Infectious endophthalmitis following sutureless cataract surgery. Arch Ophthalmol 1991;109:1562–1563
35. Ashkenazi I, Melamed S, Avni I, Bartov E. Risk factors associated with late infection of filtering blebs and endophthalmitis. Ophthalmic Surg 1991;22:570–574
36. Neuteboom GHG, De Vries-Knoppert WAEJ. Endophthalmitis after Nd:YAG laser capsulotomy. Doc Ophthalmol 1988;70:175–178
37. Javitt JC, Vitale S, Canner JK, et al. National outcomes of cataract extraction: endophthalmitis following inpatient surgery. Arch Ophthalmol 1991;109:1085–1089
38. Menikoff JA, Speaker MG, Marmor M, Raskin EM. A case-control study of risk factors for post-operative endophthalmitis. Ophthalmology 1991;98:1761–1768
39. Culver DH, Horan TC, Gaynes RP, et al. Surgical wound infection rates by wound class, operative procedure, and patient risk index. Am J Med 1991;91(suppl 3B):152S–157S
40. Maylath FR, Leopold IH. Study of experimental intraocular infection. I. The recoverability of organisms inoculated into ocular tissues and fluids. II. The influence of antibiotics and cortisone, alone and combined, on intraocular growth of these organisms. Am J Ophthalmol 1955;40:86–101

41. Christy NE, Lall P. Postoperative endophthalmitis following cataract surgery: effects of subconjunctival antibiotics and other factors. Arch Ophthalmol 1973;90: 361–366
42. Smith RJH. Endophthalmitis following cataract extraction (editorial). Br J Ophthalmol 1989;73:401
43. Jansen B, Hartmann C, Schumacher-Perdeau F, Peters G. Late onset endophthalmitis associated with intraocular lens: a case of molecularly proven *S. epidermidis* aetiology. Br J Ophthalmol 1991;75:440–441
44. Dilly PN, Holmes Sellors PJ. Bacterial adhesion to intraocular lenses. J Cataract Refract Surg 1989;15:317–320
45. Raskim E, Speaker M, Pelton-Henrion K, et al. Polypropylene haptics increase bacterial adherence to intraocular lenses (abstract). Invest Ophthalmol Vis Sci 1992;33:1420
46. Richet HM, Chidiac C, Prat A, et al. Analysis of risk factors for surgical wound infections following vascular surgery. Am J Med 1991;91(suppl 3B):170S–172S
47. Elston RA, Chattopadhyay B. Postoperative endophthalmitis. J Hosp Infect 1991; 17:243–253
48. Flynn HW Jr, Pflugfelder SC, Culbertson WW, Davis JL. Recognition, treatment and prevention of endophthalmitis. Semin Ophthalmol 1989;4(2):69–83
49. Olk RJ, Bohigian GM. The management of endophthalmitis: diagnostic and therapeutic guidelines including the use of vitrectomy. Ophthalmic Surg 1987;18: 262–267
50. Abelson MB, Allansmith MR. Normal conjunctival wound edge flora of patients undergoing uncomplicated cataract extraction. Am J Ophthalmol 1973;76:561–565
51. Mandelbaum S, Forster RK. Postoperative endophthalmitis. Int Ophthalmol Clin 1987;27:95–106
52. Hibberd PL, Schein OD, Baker AS. Intraocular infections: current therapeutic approach. In: Remington JS, Swartz MN, eds. Current clinical topics in infectious diseases, vol 11. Boston: Blackwell Scientific, 1991:118–169
53. Meredith TA, Trabelsi A, Miller MJ, et al. Spontaneous sterilization in experimental *Staphylococcus epidermidis* endophthalmitis. Invest Ophthalmol Vis Sci 1990;31: 181–186
54. Pokorny KS, Libert J, Caspers-Velu L, Goossens H. Culture-negative specimens in bacterial endophthalmitis: a new diagnostic technique using ultrasonification (abstract). Invest Ophthalmol Vis Sci 1992;33:937
55. Baum J, Peyman GA, Barza M. Intravitreal administration of antibiotic in the treatment of bacterial endophthalmitis. III. Consensus. Surv Ophthalmol 1982;26: 204–206
56. Campochiaro PA, Conway BP. Aminoglycoside toxicity: a survey of retinal specialists: implications for ocular use. Arch Ophthalmol 1991;109:946–950
57. Doft BH, Barza B. Endophthalmitis vitrectomy study (reply to letter). Arch Ophthalmol 1991;109:1061
58. Davis JL, Koidou-Tsiligianni A, Pflugfelder SC, et al. Coagulase-negative staphylococcal endophthalmitis—increase in antimicrobial resistance. Ophthalmology 1988; 95:1404–1410
59. Doft BH. The endophthalmitis vitrectomy study (editorial). Arch Ophthalmol 1991;109:487–488
60. Graham RO, Peyman GA. Intravitreal injection of dexamethasone: treatment of experimentally induced endophthalmitis. Arch Ophthalmol 1974;92:142–154
61. Huang SS, Brod RD, Flynn HW Jr. Management of endophthalmitis while preserving the uninvolved crystalline lens. Am J Ophthalmol 1991;112:695–701
62. Stern GA, Engel HM, Driebe WT Jr. The treatment of postoperative endophthalmitis: results of differing approaches to treatment. Ophthalmology 1989;96:62–67

63. Wenzel RP. Preoperative antibiotic prophylaxis. N Engl J Med 1992;326:337–339
64. Meredith TA. Prevention of postoperative infection. Arch Ophthalmol 1991;109: 944–945
65. Isenberg S, Apt L, Yoshimori R. Chemical preparation of the eye in ophthalmic surgery. II. Effectiveness of mild silver protein solution. Arch Ophthalmol 1983; 101:764–765
66. Hale LM. Povidone-iodine in ophthalmic surgery. Ophthalmic Surg 1970;1(5):9–13
67. Apt L, Isenberg SJ, Yoshimori R, Spierer A. Outpatient topical use of povidone-iodine in preparing the eye for surgery. Ophthalmology 1989;96:289–292
68. Starr MB. Prophylactic antibiotics for ophthalmic surgery. Surv Ophthalmol 1983; 27:353–373
69. Classen DC, Evans RS, Pestotnik SL, et al. The timing of prophylactic administration of antibiotics and the risk of surgical wound infection. N Engl J Med 1992;326: 281–286
70. Shockley RK, Fishman P, Aziz M, et al. Subconjunctival administration of ceftazidime in pigmented rabbit eyes. Arch Ophthalmol 1986;104:266–268

Postoperative Chronic Microbial Endophthalmitis

Sid Mandelbaum, M.D.

David M. Meisler, M.D.

In recent years, previously unsuspected microbial etiologies have been documented as causing chronic endophthalmitis after cataract extraction. The term *chronic* has been used to describe endophthalmitis that usually presents more than 1 month postoperatively and may persist for months thereafter. These temporal characteristics distinguish this entity from the more common, more virulent forms of endophthalmitis that usually occur in the immediate postoperative period.

Chronic postoperative intraocular inflammation can ensue from a variety of nonmicrobial origins or can be caused by microbial organisms. If there was no breach in the integrity of the corneoscleral wall of the eye after operation, such as occurs with a wound dehiscence, a filtering bleb, or a loose, eroded suture (and excluding the rare case of metastatic blood-borne endophthalmitis), the organisms causing the inflammatory response must have been introduced into the eye at the time of the surgical procedure. Though the focus of this chapter is primarily ocular infections, it is important to recognize the distinguishing clinical features of noninfectious causes of chronic inflammation. Epithelial downgrowth may simulate chronic postoperative endophthalmitis. The intraocularly shed epithelial cells may be misinterpreted as inflammatory cells. On careful examination, however, these clumps of epithelial cells are larger than inflammatory cells and do not respond to topical steroid therapy. Careful biomicroscopical examination may also reveal the typical glassy membrane of confluent epithelium on the iris surface, corneal endothelium, or both.

Vitreous incarceration may cause chronic postoperative inflammation, often accompanied by cystoid macular edema. In the past, intraocular lenses (IOLs) were relatively common causes of chronic endophthalmitis. With improvements in lens design, manufacture, and sterilization, inflammation caused by the intraocular lens itself is rare unless a malpositioned implant is traumatizing ocular tissue.

Inflammation induced by retained cortical or nuclear fragments is generally readily evident by history and examination. The lens-related inflammatory syndrome that has caused the greatest confusion with chronic infectious endophthalmitis has been phacoanaphylactic endophthalmitis, also called *phacoantigenic uveitis*. This entity, described early in the twentieth century and characterized by granulomatous inflammation, is considered to be an immunological response involving an abrogation of tolerance to lens protein [1] and is not dependent on the amount of retained lens material. A number of cases believed to be phacoanaphylactic endophthalmitis occurring after extracapsular cataract extraction and posterior chamber lens implantation were reported in the early to middle 1980s [2–5].

In 1986, Meisler and associates [6] reported 6 patients with chronic postoperative endophthalmitis clinically indistinguishable from phacoanaphylactic endophthalmitis, from whose vitreous or aqueous specimens these investigators were able to isolate *Propionibacterium* species, usually *P. acnes*. Since their initial report, many additional cases have been reported [7–18].

P. acnes is a gram-positive, non-spore-forming pleomorphic bacillus that is ubiquitous in nature and inhabits hair follicles and sebaceous glands of the skin. It is commonly found in the anaerobic flora of the conjunctiva [19–21]. *P. acnes* is an opportunistic pathogen that has become a recognized cause of a wide variety of infections including brain abscess, subdural empyema, parotid and dental infections, pleuropulmonary infections, peritonitis, osteomyelitis, central nervous system shunt infections, and endocarditis with and without artificial heart valves [22–25]. It has also been implicated in periocular and ocular infections such as preseptal cellulitis, canaliculitis, dacryocystitis, conjunctivitis, and keratitis [26]. *P. acnes* has been found capable of causing acute endophthalmitis after ocular trauma [27–28].

■ Clinical Features

The presentation of chronic *P. acnes* endophthalmitis in patients after cataract extraction may follow one of several patterns. In most patients, the immediate postoperative period is uneventful, with resolution of the usual mild postoperative inflammation. Weeks or months later, an affected patient may develop either gradually progressive, low-grade inflammation or an abrupt onset of severe intraocular inflammation. In a recently reported case, inflammation severe enough to decrease visual acuity from 20/30 to hand movements developed suddenly more than 2 years postoperatively [29]. Some patients with *P. acnes* endophthalmitis have developed intraocular inflammation only after neodymium–yttrium aluminum garnet (Nd:YAG) laser posterior capsulotomy, presumably due to liberation of previously loculated organisms [6, 12, 13].

The course of the inflammation in all these patterns tends to be stuttering, with exacerbations and remissions. It is usually responsive to corticosteroid therapy, at least initially. As time progresses, higher doses of corticosteroids are frequently required, often having less effect on the inflammation. If corticosteroids are tapered, inflammation may recur [30].

Patients with chronic endophthalmitis usually have both vitritis and iridocyclitis. Intraocular inflammation may be severe enough to result in a hypopyon. At some time during their course, many patients will manifest granulomatous-appearing precipitates on the corneal endothelium or on the surfaces of the IOL implant. Fibrin beaded strands across the anterior chamber have been observed in some eyes [16]. Many of the reported cases of *Propionibacterium* endophthalmitis have had a creamy white plaque or plaques present within the peripheral capsular bag or sandwiched between the IOL and the posterior capsule. Some plaques appear creamy and confluent whereas others appear more crumbly, particularly along their edges, distinguishing them from the fibrous capsular changes seen commonly after cataract extraction. These plaques may be difficult to visualize because of their peripheral location. Maximally dilating the pupil and directing the slit lamp from a very oblique angle may be helpful in observing these plaques. Histopathological studies have shown that these plaques consist of colonies of organisms, sometimes admixed with residual lens material (Fig 1).

■ Microbiological Aspects

These clinical features, though characteristic of *Propionibacterium* endophthalmitis, are not pathognomonic for infection with this organism. Definitive diagnosis of chronic postoperative inflammation with these features requires cultures of ocular specimens and particular care in processing the specimens. Because chronic endophthalmitis does not require emergent intervention, there is the opportunity to coordinate processing of the specimens with the microbiology laboratory. Once obtained, specimens should be promptly inoculated into both liquid and solid media, and the media should be incubated both aerobically and anaerobically. *P. acnes* has been isolated in thioglycolate broth and cooked meat as well as on prereduced anaerobic blood agar [30]. Cultures should be maintained for 2 weeks, because it may take this long to observe growth of certain anaerobic species. In addition to aqueous and vitreous specimens, the yield is increased if a portion of the capsular plaque itself can be cultured.

Organisms other than *Propionibacterium* that have been isolated from eyes with chronic postoperative inflammation include staphylococci (more frequently *S. epidermidis* but occasionally *S. aureus*), *Achromobacter* species, anaerobic streptococci, *Actinomyces* species, and a variety of fungi, especially *Candida* species [18, 31–34]. Anaerobes may also be found in polymicro-

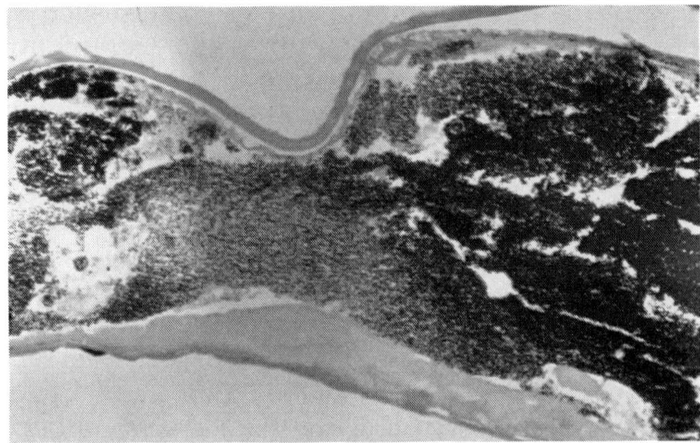

Figure 1 *Low-power light photomicrograph of confluent gram-positive pleomorphic bacilli between lens capsule remnants (tissue Gram stain).*

bial, synergistic infection with aerobic organisms. For example, both *Candida parapsilosis* and *P. acnes* have been cultured from 2 cases of chronic postoperative endophthalmitis [35]. The wide variety of organisms that can cause this clinical picture underscores the need for particularly careful cultures when surgical intervention is undertaken.

Because of the fastidious nature of many of these organisms, specimens, particularly of the excised capsule, should be examined histopathologically. If cultures are positive, histopathological demonstration of the organism in specimens of intraocular tissue verifies that the culture was not a contaminant. If there is no growth from the cultures, the presence of microbial organisms on histopathological examination may allow a presumptive diagnosis, guiding subsequent therapy. On Gram stain, *P. acnes* appears as a small, pleomorphic gram-positive bacillus. The organism has been found within inflammatory cells. By transmission electron microscopy, the organism measures 400 to 500 nm in cross-sectional diameter and up to 1,200 nm in longitudinal section. The organisms have oval, rounded, and elongated profiles, and a double cell wall. Flocculent material is seen adherent to the outer surface of the organism. The cytoplasm is variably dense and contains areas of fine stippling and dense, filamentous nuclear material [36].

■ Management Options

The optimal therapy for chronic postoperative endophthalmitis is uncertain. A wide variety of therapeutic approaches has been employed in the cases reported in the literature, with variable success. No single schema has proved universally successful. This suggests a benefit to individualizing therapy to the specific clinical circumstances, taking into account an individual's response to each therapeutic maneuver.

When a patient presents with intraocular inflammation weeks or months postoperatively, the first step remains to search diligently for any pathway through which organisms could have recently entered the eye. As previously discussed, such pathways include subtle wound dehiscences, filtering blebs, or recently removed sutures. Should any defect in the corneoscleral wall be present, the patient must be considered to have a late-onset but acute endophthalmitis, which might be caused by a virulent organism even if the presenting inflammatory manifestations are mild. Such a patient should be managed as would a patient who develops endophthalmitis in the immediate postoperative period.

Only if the corneoscleral wall is intact and there have been no recent interventions with potential for communication between the interior of the eye and the external environment can the endophthalmitis be considered to be of the chronic postoperative type discussed here. These patients, except for those in whom the clinical setting suggests a high likelihood of fungal infection, are often treated with frequent topical corticosteroids in an attempt to suppress the intraocular inflammation [30]. Although the inflammation often is suppressed initially, it usually does not resolve entirely with corticosteroid therapy.

More typically, despite corticosteroids, the inflammation gradually increases, the peripheral capsular plaque enlarges (Fig 2), and cystoid macular edema may develop. A reasonable next step in this setting would be a vitrectomy approached via the pars plana, with removal of those portions of the capsule containing the plaque. As much of the posterior capsular plaque should be removed as is possible without compromising the stability of the IOL. Use of intraocular scissors and forceps may allow excision and removal of involved portions of the posterior capsule so that they can be directly placed onto culture media. In addition to its diagnostic value, this presumably also has therapeutic benefit since the posterior capsular plaques have been identified as consisting, at least in part, of large collections of organisms. Creating an opening in the posterior capsule may also help by facilitating diffusion of antibiotics throughout the eye.

Administration of intravitreal antibiotics at the time of vitrectomy is a reasonable adjunctive measure. *P. acnes* has been shown to be sensitive to a wide spectrum of antibiotics, including cephalosporins, clindamycin, and penicillin [37, 38]. *P. acnes* recovered from ocular fluids and tissue shows similar susceptibilities based on in vitro minimum inhibitory concentration studies [39, 40]. Vancomycin is an antibiotic effective against not only *P. acnes* [41–43] but also the other gram-positive organisms that have been isolated from these cases and, at this time, appears to be the optimal choice for administration. There is little rationale for intravitreal administration of an aminoglycoside antibiotic; *P. acnes* as well as the other organisms isolated in this clinical setting are generally resistant to the aminoglycosides. If fungal organisms are identified on Gram stain, amphotericin B

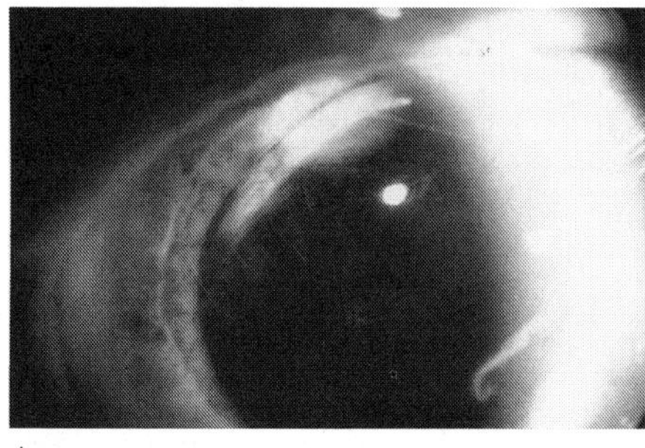

A

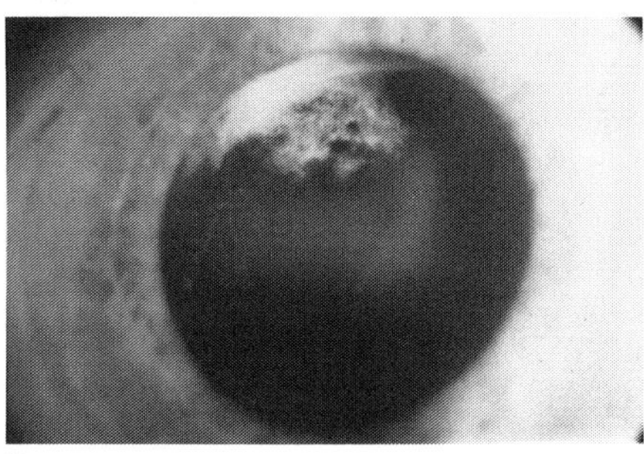

B

Figure 2 *(A) Peripheral white capsular plaque at edge of a posterior chamber lens implant in the right eye of a 75-year-old man. The patient underwent uneventful extracapsular cataract extraction and lens implantation 7 months previously. Visual acuity had been 20/30 but declined abruptly to hand movements as a result of sudden development of vitritis and iridocyclitis. Intraocular inflammation was suppressed with corticosteroids, at which time the plaque was recognized. (B) Same eye 9 months later. Low-grade inflammation was persistent, and the capsular plaque had enlarged. The patient subsequently underwent pars plana vitrectomy, excision of the posterior capsular plaque, and injection of vancomycin intraocularly. Propionibacterium acnes was cultured from the plaque and from the vitreous.*

should be injected intraocularly. Treatment failures have occurred despite intravitreal injection of appropriate antibiotics [20, 44]. One possible explanation is the slow growth rate of the *P. acnes* organism. A recent study has shown that minimum bactericidal concentration levels for some antibiotics to which *P. acnes* is usually sensitive may not uniformly kill the organism, even after 72 hours of exposure [39]. Antibiotics injected once into the vitreous cavity may not remain in sufficiently high concentrations to ensure activity during the replicative phase of the organism [45]. Another possible explanation is the apparent sequestration of organisms in the recesses of the peripheral capsule, which may insulate them from the effect of the injected antibiotics. Even if visibly involved portions of the posterior capsule have been excised, organisms may be present in other areas.

Although many patients will be cured after vitrectomy, removal of visible capsular plaques, and intravitreal antibiotic injection, some will have persistent inflammation, presumably due to residual organisms or bacterial components. If intraocular inflammation can be controlled with a low-dose regimen of topical corticosteroids, then it seems worth waiting to see whether the inflammation will resolve. If it does not, further intervention is appropriate.

Administration of oral antibiotics would seem a logical therapeutic choice in cases of *P. acnes* endophthalmitis. As noted, the organisms appear sensitive to a number of antibiotics that can be safely administered orally and that may achieve therapeutic levels within an inflamed eye. Clinical experience with oral antibiotics to date, however, has been generally disappointing, although an occasional case has been reported that may have been successfully managed in this way [14].

The procedure of final resort in these cases is removal of the implant and the entire capsular bag where organisms are presumably sequestered. This has been approached via a limbal incision. Injection of alpha-chymotrypsin may allow removal of the entire capsular bag and IOL complex, particularly if the implant was fixated within the bag. Additional vitrectomy often is required. This procedure has been effective in resolving inflammation in most cases not caused by fungi but involves more extensive surgery than vitrectomy and capsulectomy via the pars plana; it should therefore be reserved for cases wherein inflammation persists despite the measures discussed previously. Placement of an anterior chamber lens at this time has been successfully accomplished without recurrent inflammation in some patients [16].

The visual outcome in cases of chronic postoperative endophthalmitis caused by *P. acnes* or other bacterial organisms has generally been good, particularly compared to endophthalmitis that develops in the immediate postoperative period and that is caused by more virulent organisms. Persistence of chronic inflammation may result in the development of cystoid macular edema, which may not resolve entirely. Severe visual loss has been attributed to retinal detachment or to posterior vascular events.

■ Conclusion

Much remains to be learned about the nature of the organisms causing these unusual chronic postoperative inflammatory syndromes. The identification of microorganisms from these eyes has emphasized the need to be suspicious of microbial infection even in unexpected clinical settings.

■ References

1. Marak GE Jr. Phacoanaphylactic endophthalmitis. Surv Ophthalmol 1992;36: 325–339
2. Apple DJ, Mamalis N, Steinmetz RL, et al. Phacoanaphylactic endophthalmitis associated with extracapsular cataract extraction and posterior chamber intraocular lens. Arch Ophthalmol 1984;102:1528–1532
3. McMahon MS, Weiss JS, Riedel KG, Albert DM. Clinically unsuspected phacoanaphylaxis after extracapsular cataract extraction with intraocular lens implantation. Br J Ophthalmol 1985;69:836–840
4. Abrahams IW. Diagnosis and surgical management of phacoanaphylactic uveitis following extracapsular cataract extraction with intraocular lens implantation. J Am Intraocul Implant Soc 1985;11:444–447
5. Wohl LG, Lucier AC, Kline OR Jr, Galman BD. Pseudophakic phacoanaphylactic endophthalmitis. Ophthalmic Surg 1986;17:234–237

6. Meisler DM, Palestine AG, Vastine DW, et al. Chronic *Propionibacterium* endophthalmitis after extracapsular cataract extraction and intraocular lens implantation. Am J Ophthalmol 1986;102:733–739

7. Jaffe GJ, Whitcher JP, Biswell R, Irvine AR. *Propionibacterium acnes* endophthalmitis seven months after extracapsular cataract extraction and intraocular lens implantation. Ophthalmic Surg 1986;17:791–793

8. Ormerod LD, Paton BG, Haaf J, et al. Anaerobic bacterial endophthalmitis. Ophthalmology 1987;94:799–808

9. Roussel TJ, Culbertson WW, Jaffe NS. Chronic postoperative endophthalmitis associated with *Propionibacterium acnes*. Arch Ophthalmol 1987;105:1199–2001

10. Piest KL, Kincaid MC, Tetz MR, et al. Localized endophthalmitis: a newly described cause of the so-called toxic lens syndrome. J Cataract Refract Surg 1987;13:498–510

11. Meisler DM, Zakov ZN, Bruner WE, et al. Endophthalmitis associated with sequestered intraocular *Propionibacterium acnes* [letter]. Am J Ophthalmol 1987;104:428–429

12. Tetz MR, Apple DJ, Price FW Jr, et al. A newly described complication of neodymium-YAG laser capsulotomy: exacerbation of an intraocular infection [letter]. Arch Ophthalmol 1987;105:1324–1325

13. Carlson AN, Koch DD. Endophthalmitis following Nd:YAG laser posterior capsulotomy. Ophthalmic Surg 1988;19:168–170

14. Brady SE, Cohen EJ, Fischer DH. Diagnosis and treatment of chronic postoperative bacterial endophthalmitis. Ophthalmic Surg 1988;19:580–584

15. Sawusch MR, Michels RG, Stark WJ, et al. Endophthalmitis due to *Propionibacterium acnes* sequestered between IOL optic and posterior capsule. Ophthalmic Surg 1989;20:90–92

16. Zambrano W, Flynn HW Jr, Pflugfelder SC, et al. Management options for *Propionibacterium acnes* endophthalmitis. Ophthalmology 1989;96:1100–1105

17. Abrahams IW. *Propionibacterium acnes* endophthalmitis: an unusual manner of presentation. J Cataract Refract Surg 1989;15:698–701

18. Fox GM, Joondeph BC, Flynn HW Jr, et al. Delayed-onset pseudophakic endophthalmitis. Am J Ophthalmol 1991;111:163–173

19. Matuura H. Anaerobes in the bacterial flora of the conjunctival sac. Jpn J Ophthalmol 1971;15:116–124

20. Perkins RE, Kundsin RB, Pratt MV, et al. Bacteriology of normal and infected conjunctiva. J Clin Microbiol 1975;1:147–149

21. McNatt J, Allen SD, Wilson LA, Dowell VE Jr. Anaerobic flora of the normal human conjunctival sac. Arch Ophthalmol 1978;96:1448–1450

22. Johnson WD, Kaye D. Serious infections caused by diphtheroids. Ann NY Acad Sci 1970;174:568–576

23. Kamme C, Lidgren L, Lindberg L, Mardh P-A. Anaerobic bacteria in late infections after total hip arthroplasty. Scand J Infect Dis 1974;6:161–165

24. Everett ED, Eickhoff TC, Simon RH. Cerebrospinal fluid shunt infections with anaerobic diphtheroids (*Propionibacterium* species). J Neurosurg 1976;44:580–584

25. Noble RC, Overman SB. *Propionibacterium acnes* osteomyelitis: case report and review of the literature. J Clin Microbiol 1987;25:251–254

26. Smith RE, Nobe JR. Eye infections. In: Finegold SM, George WL, eds. Anaerobic infections in humans. San Diego: Academic, 1989:213–232

27. Jones DB, Robinson NM. Anaerobic ocular infections. Trans Am Acad Ophthalmol Otolaryngol 1977;83:OP309–331

28. Beatty RF, Robin JB, Trousdale MD, Smith RE. Anaerobic endophthalmitis caused by *Propionibacterium acnes* [letter]. Am J Ophthalmol 1986;101:114–116

29. Friberg TR, Kuzma PM. *Propionibacterium acnes* endophthalmitis two years after extracapsular cataract extraction [letter]. Am J Ophthalmol 1990;109:609–610

30. Meisler DM, Mandelbaum S. *Propionibacterium*-associated endophthalmitis after extracapsular cataract extraction: review of reported cases. Ophthalmology 1989; 96:54–61
31. Manka RH, Nozik RA, Stern WH. Intraocular *Staphylococcus aureus* abscess masquerading as chronic uveitis. Am J Ophthalmol 1988;105:555–556
32. Seedor JA, Koplin RS, Shah M, et al. Chronic postoperative endophthalmitis from *Staphylococcus aureus*. J Cataract Refract Surg 1990;16:512–513
33. Ficker L, Meredith TA, Wilson LA, et al. Chronic bacterial endophthalmitis. Am J Ophthalmol 1987;103:745–748
34. Roussel T, Pflugfelder S, Olson ER, et al. Delayed onset chronic postoperative endophthalmitis associated with *Actinomyces* species. Presented at the Twenty-Third Annual Meeting of the Ocular Microbiology and Immunology Group, Las Vegas, October 1988
35. Wong SK, Meisler DM, Cohen HB, et al. Chronic postoperative endophthalmitis: *Candida parapsilosis* or *Propionibacterium acnes*? Presented at the Twenty-Third Annual Meeting of the Ocular Microbiology and Immunology Group, Las Vegas, October 1988
36. Montes LF, Wilborn WH. Fine structure of *Corynebacterium acnes*. J Invest Dermatol 1970;54:338–345
37. Wang WLL, Everett ED, Johnson M, Dean E. Susceptibility of *Propionibacterium acnes* to seventeen antibiotics. Antimicrob Agents Chemother 1977;11:171–173
38. Denys GA, Jerris RC, Swenson JM, Thornsberry C. Susceptibility of *Propionibacterium acnes* clinical isolates to 22 antimicrobial agents. Antimicrob Agents Chemother 1983;23:335–337
39. Hall GS, Meisler DM, Pratt K, et al. Antibiotic susceptibility of *Propionibacterium acnes* recovered from chronic infectious endophthalmitis [ARVO abstr]. Invest Ophthalmol Vis Sci (Suppl) 1989;30:196
40. Penland R, Robinson N, Osato M. In vitro susceptibility of ocular isolates of *Propionibacterium acnes* [ARVO abstr]. Invest Ophthalmol Vis Sci (Suppl) 1989;30:197
41. Varaldo PE, Debbia E, Schito GC. In vitro activity of teichomycin and vancomycin alone and in combination with rifampin. Antimicrob Agents Chemother 1983; 23:402–406
42. Glupczynski Y, Labbe M, Crokaert F, Yourassowsky E. In vitro activity of teicoplanin and vancomycin against anaerobes. Eur J Clin Microbiol 1984;3:50–51
43. Chow AW, Cheng N. In vitro activities of daptomycin (LY146032) and paldimycin (U-70, 138F) against anaerobic gram-positive bacteria. Antimicrob Agents Chemother 1988;32:788–790
44. Stern GA, Engel HM, Driebe WT Jr. Recurrent postoperative endophthalmitis. Cornea 1990;9:102–107
45. Pflugfelder SC, Hernandez E, Fliesler SJ, et al. Intravitreal vancomycin: retinal toxicity, clearance, and interaction with gentamicin. Arch Ophthalmol 1987;105: 831–837

The Biology of Herpes Simplex and Varicella Zoster Virus Infections

Thomas J. Liesegang, M.D.

Intensive study of the biology of the herpes simplex virus (HSV) and the varicella zoster virus (VZV) and of the molecular events that occur during infection and recurrence with these viruses has yielded new information over the past decade. Knowledge about the nature of the symbiotic relationship with humans and the precise mechanisms that control recurrences may, in the future, reduce the morbidity from these ubiquitous infections.

■ General Biological Features of HSV and VZV

Both HSV and VZV are approximately 150 to 200 nm in diameter and are composed of a linear DNA and protein core, with a surrounding protein capsid, an amorphous tegument layer, and a lipid bilayer envelope (Fig 1). VZV has a slightly lower molecular weight than HSV, although the two viruses cannot be distinguished by electron microscopy. The protein capsid protects the nucleic acid and confers an icosahedral symmetry to the virus; it is important in permitting viral introduction into the host cell. The tegument is an amorphous protein structure important in inducing active viral transcription within the nucleus. The envelope of the virus is a complex phospholipoprotein structure derived from the cytoplasmic membrane of the host cell; glycoprotein subunits project from the surface of the envelope and are important in inducing a specific antibody response.

HSV and VZV are members of the subfamily alpha-herpesviruses, which are neurotrophic viruses with a capacity to establish a latent infection primarily in ganglia (Table). There are two HSV types—type I and type II—and these are antigenically related. It is still not clear why HSV type I generally involves the ocular and facial tissues, whereas HSV type II is more common in the genital area. Both primary HSV and primary VZV infections cause a systemic or disseminated infection. HSV type I is gener-

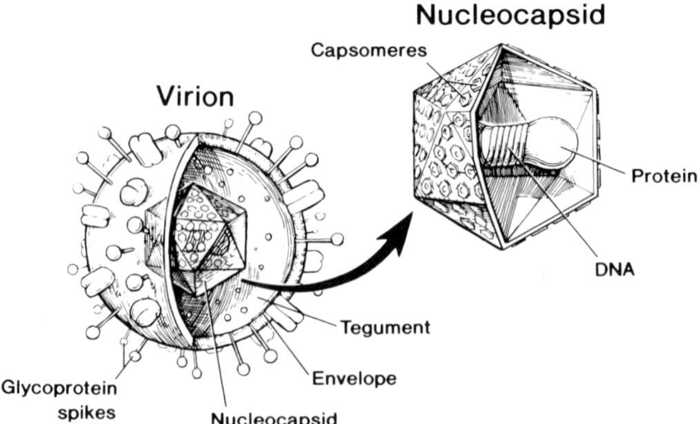

Figure 1 *Schematic drawing of a herpesvirus. The DNA genome of the herpesvirus is surrounded by protein, much like thread on a spool. A protein structure called the* capsid, *in the shape of an icosahedron, surrounds this DNA genome core. This combined structure is called a* nucleocapsid. *An additional phospholipoprotein envelope surrounds the nucleocapsid, with glycoprotein spikes projecting from the surface. The tegument is an amorphous protein structure between the nucleocapsid and envelope. The complete infectious particle is called a* virion. *(Published courtesy of Ophthalmology 1992;99: 781–799.)*

ally a childhood systemic infection that is not frequently recognized as HSV unless it presents with skin vesicles or with the typical ocular features of the virus. HSV spreads on epithelial or mucous membrane tissue and then gains access to sensory nerve endings and the ganglia. The primary infection occurs most commonly within the body surface innervated by the trigeminal nerve (i.e., the mucocutaneous areas of the face, eye, and oral mucosa), and autopsy studies reveal that 68% of patients infected with HSV harbor the viral DNA in their trigeminal ganglia [1]. Less commonly, HSV type II is present in the sacral ganglia. In immunocompromised individuals and newborns, the primary HSV infection can disseminate and be a fatal disease.

VZV is acquired through the respiratory tract and is then disseminated via the bloodstream to the skin and mucous membranes. VZV may gain access to sensory nerve endings in the skin or mucous membrane or may enter the ganglia by hematogenous spread. Primary infection with VZV involves the ganglia with acute inflammation and hemorrhagic necrosis. There is evidence of viral intranuclear bodies, VZV can be detected via electron microscopy, and the virus can be isolated during the acute phase. Viral gene products have been detected by the polymerase chain reaction in 87% of trigeminal ganglia and 55% of thoracic ganglia at autopsy in patients with a positive VZV serology [2].

Human Herpesviruses

Virus	Subgroup	Designation	Disease	Guanine and cytosine content (mol %)
Herpes simplex virus type I	Alpha	HHV 1	Oral and ocular HSV	67
Herpes simplex virus type II	Alpha	HHV 2	Genital HSV	69
Varicella zoster virus	Alpha	HHV 3	Chickenpox; herpes zoster (shingles)	46
Epstein-Barr virus	Gamma	HHV 4	Infectious mono-nucleosis	60
Human cytomegalovirus	Beta	HHV 5	Mild infection	57
Human B-cell lymphotropic virus	Beta	HHV 6	Exanthema subitum	40
Human herpesvirus 7	Beta	HHV 7	Unknown	NK

HHV = human herpesvirus; *HSV* = herpes simplex virus; *NK* = not known.

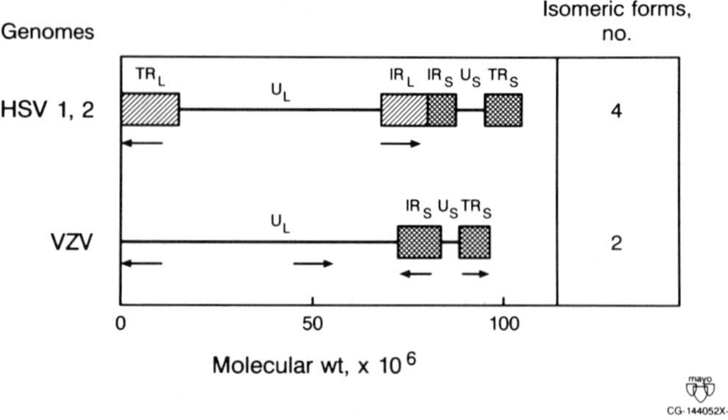

Figure 2 *Schematic drawing of the herpes simplex virus (HSV) and varicella zoster virus (VZV) genomes. Each of these viral genomes consists of long and short unique sequences (U_L, U_S), flanked by long stretches of bases that are duplicated as inverted repeat elements. These are designated as terminal or internal repeats surrounding the long and short unique sequences (TR_L, TR_S, IR_L, IR_S, respectively). Portions of the genomes that are actively transcribed in latently infected ganglia are shown as heavy arrows below the genome maps. The relative molecular weights as well as the number of isomeric forms are also depicted. (Published courtesy of Ophthalmology 1992;99:781–799.)*

Both HSV and VZV establish latency in the sensory ganglia and recur with different clinical patterns, which may be explained by their mechanisms of reactivation. Both viruses are more common in trigeminal ganglia than in other ganglia, probably because of the predominance of facial lesions during the primary infection. Although latent HSV can be isolated from trigeminal ganglia by organ culture technique, latent VZV cannot be isolated except after a recent VZV infection [3, 4].

■ The Viral Genomes

The HSV genome is approximately 152,000 base pairs and codes for approximately 72 genes and 70 different proteins [5]. The VZV genome is approximately 125,000 base pairs and codes for approximately 68 genes and 80 proteins [6]. Both viruses are composed of two portions: a unique long region and a unique short region, with gene sequences that occur only once (Fig 2). These sequences can flip-flop relative to the other, generating four possible isomeric forms of the complete DNA molecule. With HSV there are four equimolar isomers that can be extracted from infected cells, whereas VZV has two major isomers and two minor isomers. All these HSV and VZV isomers are equally infectious. The guanine and cytosine content is 67% in HSV type I, 69% in HSV type II, and 46% in VZV (see the Table). The complete genome sequences for HSV and VZV have been determined by several different techniques [5, 7]. Both viruses have similar core genes, and the sequences suggest an evolution from a common ancestor, with a series of recombinational events [6]. More extensive knowledge is available concerning HSV gene functions, and the similar genetic relationship to VZV has permitted assumption of VZV functions. The gene locations of the major glycoprotein families have been emphasized because these are important in immune recognition and, perhaps, for future vaccines. Gene analysis from clinical isolates of primary and recurrent infection have also confirmed that latent HSV and VZV reactivate [8].

Gene analysis of HSV in animal models has revealed HSV strain differences with regard to neuroinvasiveness, neurovirulence, propensity to cause corneal epithelial or stromal disease, responsiveness of ocular disease to steroids, ability to replicate in the trigeminal ganglion, and ability to reactivate endogenously or exogenously in the trigeminal ganglion or in the corneal epithelium and stroma [9–13]. Similarly, differences among animal species with regard to many aspects of HSV infection have been determined. Application of these data to humans remains speculative but is a fertile area for research [14].

■ HSV

Infection of the Neuron

The primary infection with HSV type I is generally a systemic disease with nonspecific upper respiratory symptoms. Rarely, the ocular lesions can be associated with bilateral vesicular eyelid edema, ulcerative blepharitis, or epithelial keratitis. There is initial viral replication in mucocutaneous tissue, with spread of progeny virus to contiguous cells and then to neuritic extensions of the sensory nerve. The virus attaches by surface glycoprotein spikes to receptors on the plasma membrane, with a fusion reaction [15]. Penetration of the naked viral nucleocapsids occurs, followed by a microtubular-dependent retrograde axonal flow to the nucleus at the rate of 5 to 10 mm/hr [15]. The noninfectious virion is kept structurally intact until it reaches the nucleus. When the nucleocapsid reaches the membrane of the nucleus, the viral DNA is released into the nucleus through the nuclear pore, and the empty capsid is left behind.

Within the nucleus, there is circularization of the viral DNA genome and initiation of viral replication. A coordinated and temporally related cascade of expression of three classes of genes occurs: the immediate early genes, the early genes, and the late genes (Fig 3). This ultimately results in the production of viral DNA and viral protein, which are assembled as nucleocapsids in the nucleus [16]. These nuclear inclusion bodies can be seen histologically. The host macromolecular synthesis is inhibited during this viral transcription.

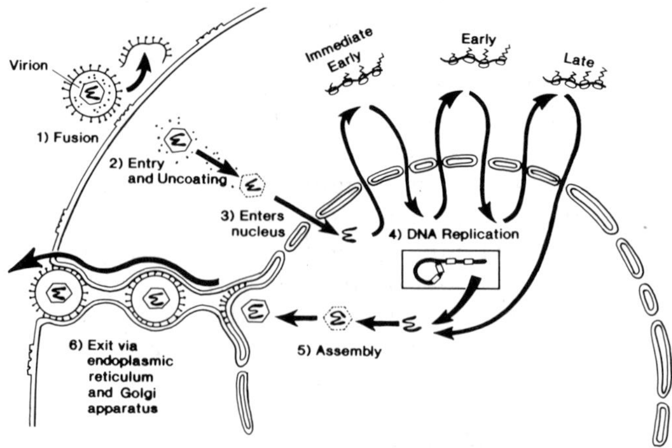

Figure 3 *Schematic replication of herpes simplex virus (HSV) in a susceptible cell. (1) The virus fuses with the plasma membrane after attachment at specific receptor sites that recognize HSV type I. The empty envelope is left at the plasma membrane. (2) The nucleocapsid is introduced into the cytoplasm and then transported to the nuclear pore by fast axoplasmic flow. Two proteins are released from the tegument of the virion. One shuts off host protein synthesis and the other is transported to the nucleus as a transducing factor (Vmw65).*
(3) The viral DNA is released into the nucleus and becomes circularized. The empty capsid coat is left at the nuclear pore. (4) In the presence of the tegument transducing factor, the transcription of the immediate early genes occurs, with transport of mRNA to the cytoplasm and translation to protein products. These products induce the transcription of early genes, with transport of mRNA to the cytoplasm and translation to beta proteins that are involved in DNA synthesis. DNA synthesis occurs by a rolling circle mechanism that yields viral DNA. Transcription of gamma genes results in the formation of gamma proteins that consist of structural proteins of the virus.
(5) The capsid proteins are constructed into complex icosahedral structures, which are packaged with viral DNA cleaved from the rolling DNA concatamers. Viral glycoprotein and tegument protein accumulate and alter the internal nuclear membrane. The nucleocapsid is probably enveloped as it passes through the internal nuclear membrane and deenveloped between the inner and outer nuclear membrane, after which it leaves the nucleus. (6) The virus is transported to the endoplasmic reticulum and Golgi apparatus, where it is enveloped and then transported via vesicles to the nerve periphery and released by exocytosis into the extracellular space or to contiguous cells. The glycoprotein spikes of the envelope are matured as the virus travels away from the nucleus. (Modified from the concepts of B. Roizman and A. E. Sears [16], and published courtesy of Ophthalmology 1992;99:781–799.)

During an active infection, the viral nucleocapsids are assembled in the cell nucleus and then enveloped at the inner lamina of the nuclear membrane. As it passes through the outer nuclear membrane, the virus is deenveloped and then again enveloped at the endoplasmic reticulum, where it becomes further enclosed in a transport vesicle. The enveloped virus is transported along the nerve in these transport vesicles for protection as well as to allow maturation of the surface glycoprotein spikes. When the virus reaches and fuses with the plasma membrane of the nerve endings, it changes the morphology and chemistry of this membrane as the virus is released by exocytosis. This host plasma membrane now contains markers that identify it for immunological attack.

Release of virus allows further infection of surrounding tissue and other nerve and satellite cells. In fact, the vesicular lesions on the skin observed in herpes simplex may not be due to multiplication of virus on the contiguous skin but rather may be the result of viral release from multiple nerve endings into a larger area of the skin (Fig 4) [17, 18]. Moreover, as an extension of this concept, the initial HSV type I infection at the orofacial site may spread up the maxillary or mandibular division to the trigeminal ganglion and, with subsequent spread of infection or at the time of reactivation, it may pass centrifugally down the ophthalmic nerve to the eye (Fig 5) [19]. Therefore, it remains unclear in humans

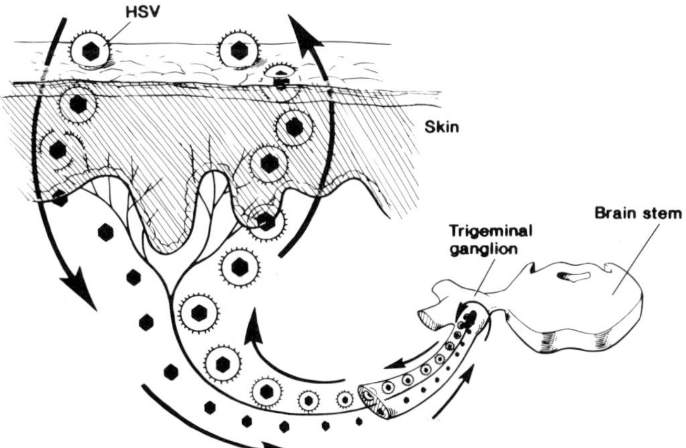

Figure 4 *The "round-trip" hypothesis of herpes simplex virus (HSV) infection. The initial replication of HSV at the inoculation site may not be essential in causing clinical disease. If the virus has access to nerve endings, it can travel as a naked nucleocapsid to the nucleus where it can undergo a replicative cycle and then travel down the nerve as an enveloped mature form. Release can then either cause the clinical lesion or at least contribute to the progression of the clinical lesion. This may explain the incubation period for clinical disease and is compatible with the "backdoor" spread of HSV. (Published courtesy of Ophthalmology 1992;99:781–799.)*

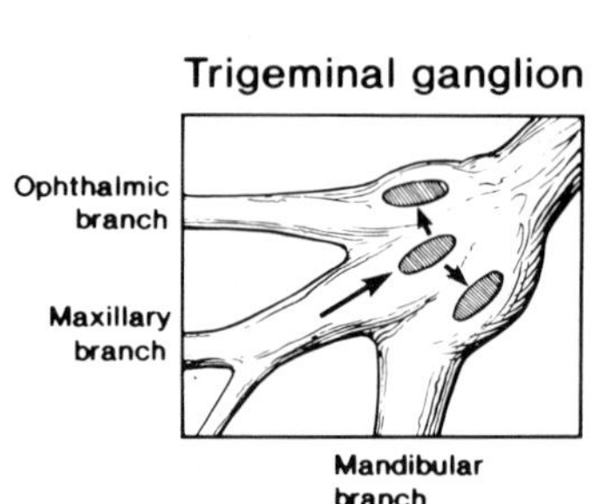
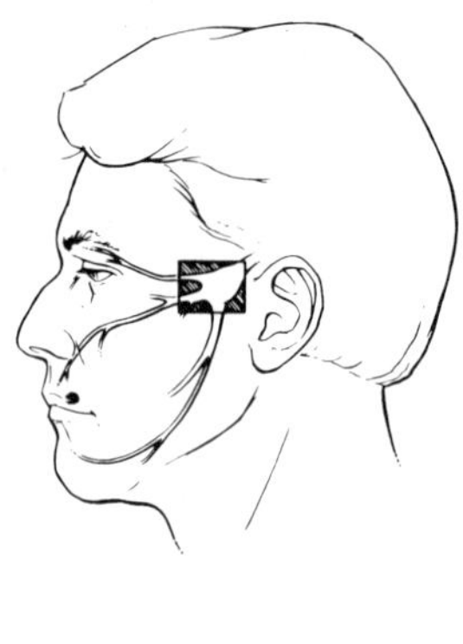

Figure 5 *The "backdoor" approach to the ophthalmic nerve causing ocular herpes simplex virus (HSV). The most common site of initial HSV infection is in the facial area served by the maxillary division of the trigeminal nerve. Infection here can result in latency in the maxillary portion of the trigeminal ganglion. At the time of initial infection, or with reactivation, virus can spread to the ophthalmic or mandibular portion of the trigeminal nerve and can perhaps cause HSV infection in the ophthalmic division of the trigeminal nerve without there ever having been a prior skin or mucous membrane HSV infection in this distribution. (Published courtesy of* Ophthalmology *1992;99:781–799.)*

whether ocular HSV infection originates from a primary ocular inoculation or whether it represents a secondary infection or reactivation descending down from the trigeminal ganglion following a prior HSV infection elsewhere in the division of the trigeminal nerve.

Cell types differ in their ability to support HSV replication. Viral replication usually results in the death of the cell, with subsequent loss of neurons. Questions linger about whether the neuron is damaged by the productive infection and whether a neuron can be the site of both a productive infection and, later, a latent infection.

Latency and Reactivation

HSV establishes latency in nerve tissues selectively, although it is not known which factors promote productive replications versus latent infection. It is hypothesized that when a viral particle reaches a neuron nucleus, either a productive replication occurs or latency develops but not both [20]. In humans, HSV DNA can be detected in 68% of trigeminal ganglia from seropositive individuals [1]. This probably relates to the high frequency and severity of HSV facial lesions. However, it is likely that fewer than 0.3% of these neurons in the trigeminal ganglia will harbor the latent virus, with probably several copies of the same viral genome in these select neurons [21]. Ganglia in close proximity probably harbor the same latent virus (if they have latent HSV), and it is unlikely that a virus can super-infect a ganglion that is already latently infected [22]. Within the human trigeminal ganglion, latent HSV is more common in the maxillary and mandibular branches compared to the ophthalmic branch, and this corre-lates with the frequency of clinical HSV. Latency in any of these three portions of the trigeminal ganglion, however, can result from a peripheral infection of any portion of the face. Latency is lifelong in a ganglion but interrupted by periodic reactivations, which may be asymptomatic or clini-cally apparent. It is not clear whether virus reactivation from the latent state results in destruction of the neuron and thus elimination of it as a source of reactivation.

The HSV genome remains phenotypically unaltered and present in its entirety during latency. It is present in a circular arrangement probably within chromatin nuclear structures and is impenetrable to the host or to antiviral therapy [23]. The events in latency are very difficult to categorize, as latency is an in vivo process and so few cells become latently infected. The establishment of latency, as opposed to a productive infection, in a cell may have to do with the simultaneous arrival at the nucleus, by axonal transport, of both the nucleocapsid and the tegument protein [20, 24]. If tegument is interrupted in its transport to the nucleus from the peripheral nerve endings, then latency ensues. The simultaneous arrival of tegument and nucleocapsid results in a productive infection. Other host factors may also interact or contribute to the establishment of latency; we know that both species and viral strain differences in rabbits affect the ability of HSV to establish latency and to reactivate [25].

During latency, HSV remains active with limited transcription of a portion of the viral genome in the nucleus of the latently infected cells [26, 27]. These latency-associated transcripts (LATs) have been a dependable marker to indicate latently infected cells in human as well as other animal systems [23, 26]. The exact role of these LATs is unknown, although they may block the expression of the early genes and protein that initiate viral replication [28]. LATs for HSV type I are common in the trigeminal gan-glion, and LATs for HSV type II are present in the sacral ganglion [29].

The exact cause of reactivation from latency is unknown, although stimuli to the ganglion, to the skin, or to both can trigger recurrences and allow an acute lytic pattern of gene expression [30]. Prostaglandins may be the final common mediator [31]. Most theories of reactivation of latent infection assume that the maintenance of the latent state is a function of cell-mediated restriction of viral infection responsive to extraneuronal stimuli [23, 32]. Stimuli act on individual neurons, producing reactivation, but not all adjacent neurons reactivate at the same time. The capacity to have repeat recurrences of HSV may depend on the number of neurons that reactivate, the fate of the neurons after viral reactivation, and the capability of sustaining a renewed neural infection or latency after each recurrent infection. It remains speculative whether reactivation encourages further latency (by providing virus to other neurons) or whether it results in a decline in recurrences (from a loss of the reactivated neuron).

■ VZV

Infection of the Neuron

Acute primary VZV infection is initiated through the respiratory route and becomes a disseminated infection via the bloodstream and lymphatics. The virus is taken up by reticuloendothelial cells and, following multiple replication cycles, a viremia occurs that causes the evident skin and mucosal vesicular lesions. The virus then gains access to sensory nerve endings and, ultimately, the sensory ganglion is infected and develops an inflammatory and hemorrhagic necrosis. Both neuronal and nonneuronal ganglion cells demonstrate acute infection, but the neuronal population is far less susceptible to VZV-induced damage compared to HSV infection [33].

Because VZV remains predominantly cell-associated throughout the virus replication cycle in vitro, it has not been possible to obtain high-titer infectious free virus. An animal model to demonstrate acute infection and latency also is not yet available. Both neuronal and glial elements demonstrate the presence of the VZV genome during acute infection in model systems [4]. During active infection in both neuronal and nonneuronal cells, there appears to be a sequential and temporal transcription of genes with a mechanism probably similar to HSV replication.

Latency

Unlike HSV, attempts to coculture VZV from the trigeminal ganglion have been unsuccessful unless there has been a recent VZV infection. The activity of VZV genes, however, has been detected in 87% of trigeminal ganglia and 53% of thoracic ganglia of seropositive individuals [2]. The latent VZV appears to be harbored in nonneuronal cells [34], compared to HSV latency in neuronal cells. Only approximately 0.01 to 0.15% of nonneuronal cells exhibit VZV latency. Therefore, although the initial active infection with VZV appears to involve both neuronal and nonneuronal cells, during latency, VZV genome activity appears to be limited to nonneuronal cells. This persistence of VZV in nonneuronal cells may explain the facilitation of VZV spread following reactivation, with the more widespread cutaneous involvement seen in zoster, compared to the more limited cutaneous involvement after HSV reactivation [34]. The nonneuronal location of VZV latency may also explain the infrequency of VZV reactivation compared to HSV reactivation since VZV is removed from neuronal triggers [34]. Several immunological evaluations in humans [37] confirm that frequent reactivations of VZV occur but remain contained by cell-mediated immunity and that the dermatological lesions and associated dissemination of zoster occur only when this cell-mediated immunity is depressed.

■ Corneal Latency of HSV and VZV

Viral latency in the cornea is an extremely complex subject. Many studies have provided fragments of the puzzle that, once completed, may prove this hypothesis [35]. Electron microscopy, biochemical studies, and coculture studies have supported the concept of corneal viral latency and, after review of available data, Cook and Hell [36] suggested that 0 to 30% of corneas may exhibit HSV latency compared to 100% of trigeminal ganglia. Latency of HSV in nonneuronal cells (such as the cornea) is conceivable and consistent with a probable nonneuronal latency of VZV. The role of corneal latency in the different clinical HSV conditions of necrotizing stromal keratitis, disciform keratitis, and chronic stromal interstitial keratitis is not resolved, and proving such latency may alter our therapeutic strategies. The concept of latency in corneal tissue is disturbing to eye banks, although it has never been demonstrated to be clinically significant.

Latency of VZV in the cornea also is conceivable, especially since VZV appears to prefer nonneuronal cells during latency. Nonetheless, laboratory investigational studies of VZV lag well behind those of HSV and will continue to do so until a reproducible animal model can be developed.

This work was presented in part at the Annual Meeting of the American Academy of Ophthalmology, Anaheim, CA, October 13–17, 1991, and was published previously in *Ophthalmology* under the title, "Biology and Molecular Aspects of Herpes Simplex and Varicella-zoster Virus Infections," 1992;99:781–799.

■ References

1. Efstathiou S, Minson C, Field JH, et al. Detection of herpes simplex virus–specific DNA sequences in latently infected mice and humans. J Virol 1986;57:446–455
2. Mahalingram R, Wellish M, Wolf W, et al. Latent varicella zoster viral DNA in human trigeminal and thoracic ganglia. N Engl J Med 1990;323:627–631
3. Ostrove JM. Molecular biology of varicella zoster virus. Adv Virus Res 1990;38:45–97
4. Pavan-Langston D, Dunkel EC. Ocular varicella-zoster virus infection in the guinea pig. Arch Ophthalmol 1989;107:1068–1072
5. McGeoch DJ, Dalrymple MA, Davison AJ, et al. The complete sequence of the long unique region in the genome of herpes simplex virus type 1. J Gen Virol 1988;69:1531–1574
6. Davison AJ. Varicella-zoster virus. J Gen Virol 1991;72:475–486

7. Davison AJ, Scott JE. The complete DNA sequences of varicella-zoster virus. J Gen Virol 1986;67:1759–1816

8. Straus SE, Reinhold W, Smith HA, et al. Endonuclease analysis of viral DNA from varicella and subsequent zoster infection in the same patient. N Engl J Med 1984;311:1362–1364

9. Stulting RD, Kindle JC, Nahmias AJ. Patterns of herpes simplex keratitis in inbred mice. Invest Ophthalmol Vis Sci 1985;26:1360–1367

10. Stevens JG. Defining herpes simplex genes involved in neurovirulence and neuroinvasiveness. Curr Eye Res 1987;6:63–67

11. Centifanto-Fitzgerald YM, Yamaguchi T, Kaufman HE, et al. Ocular disease pattern induced by herpes simplex is genetically determined by a specific region of viral DNA. J Exp Med 1982;155:475–489

12. Kaufman HE, Varnell ED, Centifanto YM, Kessling GE. Effect of the herpes simplex virus genome on the response of infection to corticosteroids. Am J Ophthalmol 1985;100:114–118

13. Hill JA, Rayfield MA, Haruta Y. Strain specificity of spontaneous and adrenergically induced HSV-1 ocular reactivation in latently infected rabbits. Curr Eye Res 1987;6:91–97

14. Rinne JR, Abghari SZ, Stulting RD. The severity of herpes simplex viral keratitis in mice does not reflect the severity of disease in humans. Invest Ophthalmol Vis Sci 1992;33:268–272

15. Lycke E, Hamark B, Johansson M, et al. Herpes simplex virus infection of the human sensory neuron. An electron microscopy study. Arch Virol 1988;101:87–104

16. Roizman B, Sears AE. An inquiry into the mechanisms of herpes simplex virus latency. Annu Rev Microbiol 1987;4:543–571

17. Klein R. Problems of herpes virus latency. Antiviral Res 1985;1(S):111–120

18. Klein RJ. Pathogenic mechanisms of recurrent herpes simplex viral infections. Arch Virol 1976;51:1–13

19. Tullo AB, Shimeld C, Blyth WA, et al. Spread of virus and distribution of latent infection following ocular herpes simplex in the non-immune and immune mouse. J Gen Virol 1982;63:95–101

20. Steiner I, Spivack JG, Deshmane SL, et al. A herpes simplex virus type I mutant containing a nontransducing Vmw 65 protein establishes latent infection in vivo in the absence of viral replication and reactivates efficiently from explanted trigeminal ganglia. J Virol 1990;64:1630–1638

21. Green MT, Knesek JE, Dunkel EC, et al. Localization of ^{3}H-thymidine-labeled HSV-I in latently infected rabbit trigeminal ganglion cells. Invest Ophthalmol Vis Sci 1987;28:394–397

22. Centifanto-Fitzgerald YM, Varnell ED, Kaufman HE. Initial herpes simplex virus Type I infection prevents ganglionic superinfection by other strains. Infect Immun 1982;35:1125

23. Fraser NW, Spivack JG, Wroblewska Z, et al. A review of the molecular mechanisms of HSV-I latency. Curr Eye Res 1991;10(S):1–13

24. Roizman B, Sears AE. Herpes simplex viruses and their replication. In: Fields BN, Knipe DM, eds. Virology, ed 2. New York: Raven Press, 1990:1795–1841

25. Gordon YJ. Pathogenesis and latency of herpes simplex virus type 1 (HSV-1): an ophthalmologist's view of the eye as a model for the study of the virus-host relationship. Adv Exp Med Biol 1990;278:205–209

26. Croen KD, Ostrove JM, Dragovic LJ, et al. Latent herpes simplex virus in human trigeminal ganglia: detection of an intermediate-early gene "antisense" transcript by in situ hybridization. N Engl J Med 1987;317:1427–1432

27. Stevens JG, Wagner EK, Devi-Rao GB, et al. RNA complementary to a herpesvirus

and gene-in RNA is prominent in latently infected neurons. Science 1987;235: 1056–1059

28. Latchman DS. Current status review: molecular biology of herpes simplex virus latency. J Exp Pathol 1990;71:133–144
29. Croen KD, Ostrove JM, Dragovic L, Straus SE. Characterization of herpes simplex virus type 2 latency-associated transcription in human sacral ganglia and in cell culture. J Infect Dis 1991;163:23–28
30. Hill TJ. Herpes simplex virus latency. In: Roizman B, ed. The herpesvirus, vol 3. New York: Plenum, 1985:175–240
31. Yates F, Centifanto YM, Caldwell DR. The effect of modulating the synthesis and arachidonic acid cascade products on HSV lesion recurrence. Curr Eye Res 1987;6:99–104
32. Lycke E. Biological and molecular aspects on herpes simplex virus latency. Scand J Infect Dis 1990;69(S):113–119
33. Wigdahl B, Rong BL, Kinney-Thomas E. Varicella-zoster virus infection of human sensory neurons. Virology 1986;152:384–399
34. Croen KD, Ostrove JM, Dragovic LJ, Straus SE. Patterns of gene expression and sites of latency in human ganglia are different for varicella-zoster and herpes simplex viruses. Proc Natl Acad Sci USA 1988;85:9773–9777
35. Gordon UG, Romanowski E, Araullo-Cruz T, McKnight JLC. HSV-I corneal latency (letter to editor). Invest Ophthalmol Vis Sci 1991;32:663–665
36. Cook SD, Hell JH. Herpes simplex virus: molecular biology and the possibility of corneal latency. Surv Ophthalmol 1991;36:140–148
37. Liesegang TJ. Diagnosis and therapy of herpes zoster ophthalmicus. Ophthalmology 1991;98:1216–1229

Ophthalmic Manifestations of Epstein-Barr Virus Infection

Stephen C. Pflugfelder, M.D.

Cecelia A. Crouse, Ph.D.

Sally S. Atherton, Ph.D.

Epstein-Barr virus (EBV) is a ubiquitous herpesvirus that infects the majority of humans by early adulthood [1]. The virus is capable of establishing latency in mucosa-associated lymphoid tissue (MALT) [1, 2], of which the human lacrimal gland and conjunctiva are components. Over the last decade, there has been increasing recognition that EBV may be involved in the pathogenesis of ocular inflammatory diseases that develop at the time of primary EBV infection or result from reactivation of latent virus [3]. The association between EBV and certain ocular diseases has been directly established by serological tests confirming acute primary infection or by culturing the virus from, or detecting virus-associated antigens or genomes in, involved ocular tissues. In other ocular diseases, the association has been made by detecting elevated EBV serum antibody titers consistent with chronic or persistent infection; the role of EBV in the pathogenesis of these diseases is less clear. Current knowledge regarding EBV infection of ocular MALT and the association of EBV with external ocular, retinal, uveal, and neuroophthalmological disease is reviewed herein.

■ Persistent EBV Infection in Ocular MALT

EBV is capable of infecting B lymphocytes and epithelial cells in humans [1]. EBV infection of B lymphocytes occurs by binding of EBV envelope glycoprotein gp350/220 to a cell membrane protein, CD21, which also functions as the receptor for the C3d complement fragment [4]. The role of CD21 as a receptor for EBV infection of epithelial cells has not been firmly established, although one preliminary study reported that attachment of EBV to cultured epithelial cells was significantly reduced by pretreatment with anti-CD21 antibodies [5]. Levine and associates [6] reported that human lacrimal gland ductal and suprabasal conjunctival and corneal epithelia showed strong immunoreactivity with anti-CD21 antibodies.

EBV has been reported to persist in human MALT after primary infection [7, 8]. Using the sensitive in vitro DNA amplification technique, the polymerase chain reaction, EBV genomes were amplified in 10% of normal corneal epithelia [7] and 32% of normal lacrimal gland biopsies [8]. Intralobular duct epithelia were recently identified as the sites of persistent EBV infection in human lacrimal glands by in situ DNA hybridization. EBV infection in these glands was found to be limited to a small percentage of intralobular ducts. Persistent EBV infection in human lacrimal glands appears to be in a latent nonpathological state, because no EBV antigens have been detected in normal lacrimal glands [Crouse and associates, unpublished manuscript] and no EBV shedding into the tears has been detected in asymptomatic EBV-seropositive individuals [9]. Interestingly, ductal epithelia have also been reported to be the cellular sites of EBV persistence in normal human parotid and labial salivary glands [10–12].

■ External Ocular Diseases

Ocular Manifestations of Infectious Mononucleosis

Numerous cases of conjunctivitis occurring in patients with infectious mononucleosis (IM) syndrome were reported prior to the availability of specific tests to confirm a clinical diagnosis of IM [13]. More recently, external ocular manifestations of systemic EBV infection have been reported in patients with serologically confirmed IM. In 1981, Meisler and colleagues [14] reported a case of a unilateral conjunctival inflammatory mass and an enlarged preauricular lymph node in an 11-year-old boy with acute IM. The conjunctival lesion was biopsied, and an intense lymphocytic infiltrate with occasional multinucleate giant cells was observed in histological sections. Wilhelmus [15] reported a case of unilateral keratoconjunctivitis in a 16-year-old girl with acute IM. A follicular conjunctivitis and preauricular lymph node were noted in this patient, and EBV was cultured from her tears and conjunctiva. Matoba and associates [16] also noted conjunctival inflammation consisting of mild hyperemia, occasionally accompanied by a follicular tarsal conjunctival response, in a series of patients with IM and concurrent ocular anterior segment inflammation. Gardner and co-workers [17] recently reported a case of a bulbar conjunctival nodule associated with unilateral enlarged preauricular and submandibular lymph nodes in a 38-year-old patient with acute IM. Mature lymphocytes and plasma cells were noted in histological sections, and scattered cells in the lesion stained positively for EBV-associated antigens (latent membrane protein and nuclear antigen 2).

EBV has been implicated as a causative agent of both epithelial and stromal keratitis. Multiple small corneal epithelial dendrites involving the central and peripheral cornea were reported to occur in a patient with IM [15]. Several types of corneal stromal keratitis have been observed in patients with IM, including multiple focal anterior subepithelial infiltrates similar to those occurring in adenoviral infection [18], multiple granular ring-shaped or nummular opacities scattered throughout the anterior or midstroma [16, 19], and middle to deep peripheral stromal infiltrates with vascularization [16]. Pflugfelder and associates [20] recently identified EBV lytic-cycle antigens (EA-R, EA-D) and EBV DNA in cells from small corneal epithelial dendrites that recurred over a several-year period following a chemical facial peel. The solution used for chemoexfoliation in this patient contained phorbol esters, chemicals that in nanogram concentrations are capable of inducing viral replication in B lymphocytes latently infected with EBV. This patient developed pleomorphic ring-shaped infiltrates in the anterior stroma, similar to those previously reported in IM patients [16], underlying several of the epithelial lesions. The consistent morphology of the epithelial and stromal lesions observed during acute or reactivated EBV infection suggests that EBV is capable of infecting corneal epithelium and that this virus may be an agent responsible for dendritic epithelial lesions from which herpes simplex virus cannot be demonstrated [7]. Similar to other herpesviruses, EBV also appears capable of inducing stromal keratitis.

Iridocorneal Endothelial Syndrome

Tsai and colleagues [21] recently reported the association of elevated EBV viral capsid antibodies (VCA) in patients with iridocorneal endothelial (ICE) syndrome. Because lymphocytic infiltration of the endothelium has been observed histologically in corneal buttons obtained from patients with ICE syndrome [22], Tsai and co-workers [21] postulated that the corneal endothelial disease in patients with the ICE syndrome may be due to EBV infection of the endothelium. To date, the endothelium in corneal buttons removed from patients with ICE syndrome who require corneal transplantation have not been evaluated for the presence of EBV to confirm this hypothesis.

Ocular Manifestations of Sjögren's Syndrome

EBV has been implicated as a pathogenic agent in Sjögren's syndrome (SS), an immunological disease that affects MALT. The pathological changes observed in ocular MALT in SS patients include lacrimal gland lymphoproliferation consisting of B cells and CD4$^+$ T lymphocytes [23], replacement or destruction of glandular secretory acinar and ductal epithelia [24], and conjunctival squamous metaplasia, goblet cell loss, and mucous aggregate formation [25]. There is increasing clinical and laboratory evidence to support the association of EBV and SS. There have been several reported cases of primary SS developing immediately after serologically confirmed IM [26–28]. Many of the mucosal sites commonly involved in SS, such as the salivary glands, oropharynx, and cervix, are also sites of EBV persistence after primary infection [1]. Benign lymphoepithelial lesions (epimyoepithelial islands), which are frequently observed in SS lacrimal gland biopsies, have histological characteristics similar to those observed in undifferentiated nasopharyngeal and thymic carcinomas, which have been reported to contain EBV genomes [24]. Elevated serum antibody titers to EBV viral capsid and early antigens consistent with chronic EBV infection have been detected in SS patients [29, 30]. SS-B (La) antibodies, which are occasionally detected in the sera of SS patients [24], precipitate nonhistone nuclear proteins complexed with EBERs, one of the most abundant mRNA transcripts in EBV growth-transformed B cells.

Recently, EBV genomic sequences have been amplified by the polymerase chain reaction in a statistically greater percentage of peripheral blood mononuclear cell specimens, tears, and salivary and lacrimal gland biopsies of SS patients than normal controls [9, 31]. By in situ DNA hybridization, EBV genomes were detected in the majority of intralobular and interlobular ducts as well as in mononuclear cells in areas of B lymphoproliferation in 86% of SS lacrimal glands. In all SS lacrimal glands evaluated, several different EBV lytic-cycle antigens were detected in ductal epithelia and mononuclear cells in areas of B lymphoproliferation [Pflugfelder and associates, unpublished report].

The experimental data thus far suggest that EBV may play a significant role in the lacrimal gland B-cell proliferation and epithelial cell pathology observed in SS [9]. In normal patients, EBV-induced B-cell proliferation in MALT is most likely prevented by a competent cellular immune system. Risk factors for SS such as female gender, HLA type [32], and cellular immune dysfunction [9, 29] may predispose to B-cell proliferation in the lacrimal gland and other MALT as a result of poor immunosuppression of latent EBV-infected cells. The precise role, if any, that these various risk factors play in the development of ocular MALT pathology in SS remains to be elucidated.

■ Neuroophthalmological, Retinal, and Uveal Diseases

Neuroophthalmological and ocular posterior segment diseases have been reported in patients with clinical or serological evidence of IM. In

1952, Tanner [13] reviewed several cases of unilateral or bilateral optic neuritis, occasionally accompanied by retinal edema, occurring in patients in whom a clinical diagnosis of IM had been made that, in some cases, was confirmed by detection of heterophile antibodies. More recently, a case of severe optic neuritis in a patient with serologically confirmed IM was reported by Jones and associates [33]. Ophthalmoplegia due to single or multiple palsies of cranial nerves III, IV, and VI, as well as Bell's palsy, has been observed in patients with IM [34, 35].

Retinitis was found in 2 patients in whom IM was diagnosed clinically and serologically. This manifested as a deep punctate retinitis in one patient [36] and as full-thickness retinitis in the other [37]. Both these patients also had detectable serum antibodies to *Toxoplasma gondii,* and both received systemic treatment for this infectious agent.

Mild nongranulomatous anterior uveitis has been observed in several patients with IM [13]. More recently, Wong and co-workers [38] reported bilateral anterior uveitis in 2 patients with acute IM. One of these patients had bilateral papilledema, and the other had peripheral corneal edema with multiple, confluent geographical patches of white keratic precipitates underlying the stromal edema. In the same article, these authors reported a case of bilateral panuveitis in a patient with markedly elevated EBV serum antibodies consistent with a chronic infection [38]. In 1987, Tiedeman [39] reported a syndrome of multifocal choroiditis, pigment epithelial disturbance, and vitritis in patients with chronically elevated EBV viral capsid antigen IgM and early antigen titers. Recently, Usui and associates [40] have postulated that EBV may play a role in the pathogenesis of Vogt-Koyanagi-Harada syndrome because they were able to detect EBV genomic sequences in 75% of cerebrospinal fluid specimens from Vogt-Koyanagi-Harada syndrome patients but not in cerebrospinal fluid specimens from patients with other diseases.

■ Conclusion

Clinical and laboratory data suggest that EBV may be directly or indirectly involved in the pathogenesis of a variety of ocular diseases. In some cases, the association between EBV and certain ocular diseases has only recently been recognized, and additional research will be required to establish the exact pathogenic role of EBV.

This work was supported in part by Public Health Service research grants EY08711 (SCP) and EY06012 (SSA), training grant EY07021 (CAC), and core grant EY02180, through the National Institutes of Health, National Eye Institute, Bethesda, MD.

■ References

1. Rickinson AB. On the biology of Epstein-Barr virus persistence: a reappraisal. In: Lopez C, ed. Immunobiology and prophylaxis of herpesvirus infections. New York: Plenum, 1990:137–146
2. Klein G. Viral latency and transformation: the strategy of Epstein-Barr virus. Cell 1989;58:5–8
3. Matoba AY. Ocular disease associated with Epstein-Barr virus infection. Surv Ophthalmol 1990;35:145–150
4. Fingeroth JD, Weiss JJ, Tedder TF, et al. Epstein-Barr virus receptor of human B-lymphocytes in the C3d receptor of CR2. Proc Natl Acad Sci USA 1984;81:4510–4515
5. Sixbey JN. Epstein-Barr virus and epithelial cells. In: Klein G, ed. Advances in viral oncology, vol 8. New York: Raven, 1989:187–202
6. Levine J, Pflugfelder SC, Yen M, et al. Detection of the complement (CD21)/EBV receptor in human lacrimal gland and ocular surface epithelia. Reg Immunol 1990/1991;3:164–170
7. Crouse CA, Pflugfelder SC, Pereira I, et al. Detection of herpes viral genomes in normal and diseased corneal epithelium. Curr Eye Res 1990;9:569–581
8. Crouse CA, Pflugfelder SC, Cleary T, et al. Detection of Epstein-Barr virus genomes in normal human lacrimal glands. J Clin Microbiol 1990;28:1026–1032
9. Pflugfelder S, Crouse C, Pereira I, Atherton S. Amplification of Epstein-Barr virus genomic sequences in blood cells, lacrimal glands, and tears from primary Sjogren's syndrome patients. Ophthalmology 1990;97:976–984
10. Wolf H, Haus M, Wilmes E. Persistence of Epstein-Barr virus in the parotid gland. J Virol 1984;51:795–798
11. Mariette X, Golzan J, Clerc D, et al. Detection of Epstein-Barr virus DNA by in situ hybridization and polymerase chain reaction in salivary gland biopsies from patients with Sjogren's syndrome. Am J Med 1991;90:286–294
12. Venables PJW, Teo CG, Baboonian C, et al. Persistence of Epstein-Barr virus in salivary gland biopsies from healthy individuals and patients with Sjogren's syndrome. Clin Exp Immunol 1989;75:359–364
13. Tanner OR. Ocular manifestations of infectious mononucleosis. Arch Ophthalmol 1952;51:229–241
14. Meisler DM, Bosworth DE, Krachmer JH. Ocular infectious mononucleosis manifested as Parinaud's oculoglandular syndrome. Am J Ophthalmol 1981;92:722–726
15. Wilhelmus KR. Ocular involvement in infectious mononucleosis. Am J Ophthalmol 1981;91:117–118
16. Matoba AY, Wilhelmus KR, Jones DB. Epstein-Barr viral stromal keratitis. Ophthalmology 1986;93:746–751
17. Gardner BP, Margolis TP, Mondino BJ. Conjunctival lymphocytic nodule associated with the Epstein-Barr virus. Am J Ophthalmol 1991;112:567–571
18. Matoba AY, Jones DB. Corneal subepithelial infiltrates associated with systemic Epstein-Barr viral infection. Ophthalmology 1987;94:1669–1671
19. Pinnolis M, McCulley JP, Urman JD. Nummular keratitis associated with infectious mononucleosis. Am J Ophthalmol 1980;89:791–794
20. Pflugfelder S, Huang A, Crouse C. Epstein-Barr keratitis after a chemical facial peel. Am J Ophthalmol 1990;110:572–573
21. Tsai CS, Ritch R, Strauss SE, et al. Antibodies to Epstein-Barr virus in iridocorneal endothelial syndrome. Arch Ophthalmol 1990;108:1572–1576
22. Alvarado JA, Murphy CG, Juster RP, Hetherington J. Pathogenesis of Chandler's syndrome, essential iris atrophy and the Cogan-Reese syndrome. II: Estimated age at disease onset. Invest Ophthalmol Vis Sci 1986;27:873–882

23. Pepose JS, Akata RF, Pflugfelder SC, Voight W. Mononuclear cell phenotypes and immunoglobulin gene rearrangements in lacrimal gland biopsies from patients with Sjogren's syndrome. Ophthalmology 1990;97:1599–1605
24. Pflugfelder SC, Wilhelmus KR, Osato MS, et al. The autoimmune nature of aqueous tear deficiency. Ophthalmology 1986;93:1513–1517
25. Pflugfelder SC, Huang AJW, Feuer W, et al. Conjunctival cytologic features of primary Sjogren's syndrome. Ophthalmology 1990;97:985–991
26. Whittingham S, McNeilage J, Mackay I. Primary Sjogren's syndrome after infectious mononucleosis. Ann Intern Med 1985;102:490–493
27. Pflugfelder S, Roussel T, Culbertson W. Primary Sjogren's syndrome after infectious mononucleosis. JAMA 1987;257:1049–1050
28. Gaston JSH, Rowe M, Bacon P. Sjogren's syndrome after infection by Epstein-Barr virus. J Rheumatol 1990;17:558–561
29. Pflugfelder SC, Tseng SCG, Pepose JS, et al. Epstein-Barr virus infection and immunologic dysfunction in patients with aqueous tear deficiency. Ophthalmology 1990;97:313–323
30. Yamaoka K, Miyasaka N, Yamamoto K. Possible involvement of Epstein-Barr virus in the polyclonal B cell activation in Sjogren's syndrome. Arthritis Rheum 1988; 31:1014–1021
31. Saito I, Compton T, Fox RI. Detection of Epstein-Barr virus DNA by polymerase chain reaction in blood and tissue biopsies from patients with Sjogren's syndrome. J Exp Med 1989;169:2191–2198
32. Moutsopoulos H, Mann D, Johnson A, Chused T. Genetic differences between primary and secondary sicca symptoms. N Engl J Med 1979;301:761–763
33. Jones J, Gardner W, Newman T. Severe optic neuritis in infectious mononucleosis. Ann Emerg Med 1988;17:361–364
34. Davie CJ, Ceballos R, Little SC. Infectious mononucleosis with fatal neuronitis. Arch Neurol 1963;9:71–78
35. Grose C, Henle W, Henle G, Feorine PM. Primary Epstein-Barr virus infections in acute neurologic diseases. N Engl J Med 1975;292:392–395
36. Raymond LA, Wilson CA, Linnemann CC, et al. Punctate outer retinitis in acute Epstein-Barr virus infection. Am J Ophthalmol 1987;104:424–425
37. Kelly SP, Rosenthal AR, Nicholson KG, Woodard CG. Retinochoroiditis in acute Epstein-Barr virus infection. Br J Ophthalmol 1989;73:1002–1003
38. Wong KW, D'Amico DJ, Hedges TR, et al. Ocular involvement associated with chronic Epstein-Barr virus disease. Arch Ophthalmol 1987;105:788–792
39. Tiedeman JS. Epstein-Barr viral antibodies in multifocal choroiditis and panuveitis. Am J Ophthalmol 1987;103:659–663
40. Usui N, Usui N, Goto H, et al. Detection of Epstein-Barr virus DNA by polymerase chain reaction in cerebrospinal fluid from patients with Vogt-Koyanagi-Harada disease. Invest Ophthalmol Vis Sci 1991;32:807

Ocular Infections in the Acquired Immunodeficiency Syndrome

Pravin U. Dugel, M.D.
Narsing A. Rao, M.D.

The human suffering caused by the acquired immunodeficiency syndrome (AIDS) is enormous. AIDS is a universally fatal disease that usually affects people in the prime of their lives. Unfortunately, despite efforts to control its spread, the incidence of the disease continues to increase. Between December 1989 and November 1990, a total of 42,442 AIDS cases in the United States and its territories were reported to the Centers for Disease Control (CDC), which represented an annual rate of 16.7 cases per 100,000 population [1]. Between December 1988 and November 1989, 35,614 AIDS cases were reported, representing an annual rate of 14.1% [1]. These data show a 9% increase from 1988 to 1989 [2]. The cumulative total number of AIDS cases reported through November 1990 was 157,525 [3].

The number of individuals who were seropositive for the human immunodeficiency virus (HIV) is much more difficult to establish, though undoubtedly is far greater. As of 1988, the estimated number of seropositive individuals ranged from 400,000 to 2 million [4]. A study conducted in a sexually transmitted disease clinic in New Mexico found an overall male seropositivity rate of 2.4%, whereas the rate in the male homosexual and bisexual population was 14.33% [5]. The homosexual and bisexual population continues to have the greatest prevalence of seropositivity, ranging from 10 to 70% [6]. This group accounts for 50% of all reported cases of AIDS [1, 2]. Other high-risk groups include intravenous drug users and hemophiliacs.

The role of the ophthalmologist in diagnosing and managing patients with AIDS is becoming increasingly important. Ocular manifestations have been reported in up to 70% of AIDS patients [7]. It is becoming increasingly apparent that these ocular manifestations reflect systemic disease and sometimes may be the first sign of a disseminated systemic infection [7]. Therefore, in patients with AIDS, the ophthalmologist has the opportunity to make not only a sight-saving but indeed a lifesaving diagnosis. The systemic infections that involve the eye include cytomegalovirus (CMV), *Pneumocystis carinii, Cryptococcus neoformans, Mycobacterium avium-intracellulare, Candida* species, and others. Such infections can involve the ocular adnexa, anterior segment, or posterior segment, but visual morbidity is seen most often with posterior segment involvement.

■ Posterior Segment Infections

Several infectious agents—among them CMV, *C. neoformans,* and *P. carinii*—involve the retina, choroid, and optic nerve. Most posterior segment infections are from one of these sources.

CMV Retinitis

CMV retinitis is the most common opportunistic ocular infection in patients with AIDS, occurring in 15 to 40% [7–13]. In a retrospective study of 100 AIDS patients with CMV retinitis, the median time between diagnosis of AIDS and the development of CMV retinitis was 9 months [14]. It is estimated that 20,000 new cases of CMV retinitis will be reported in the United States in 1992 [15, 16].

Disease Characteristics and Clinical Findings   The modes of transmission for CMV are not completely understood, although epidemiological and virological studies implicate close or intimate contact with individuals shedding virus in urine, saliva, or other excretions [17]. Venereal transmission is believed to be the major source of infection in homosexual and bisexual individuals. CMV infection in the normal adult and in children is asymptomatic but can occasionally be associated with a mononucleosislike syndrome. In infected individuals, chronic viral shedding may occur in the urine or oral secretions. Moreover, after the primary infection, CMV is capable of establishing a latent viral infection in which the genome persists in cells but the virus itself cannot be detected by conventional culture. In contrast to the generally benign course of CMV infection in healthy individuals, CMV represents a major cause of morbidity and mortality in patients who are immunocompromised.

Well-established CMV retinitis is easily recognized as a full-thickness granular retinal opacification with hard exudates and hemorrhages. Often there is an abrupt transition between areas of necrotic retina and normal-appearing retina. The infection usually spreads along one of the major vascular arcades (Fig 1). Due to the severe immunosuppression, there is minimal overlying vitreous inflammation. The retinitis often starts in an area of a preexisting cotton-wool spot. Very early in its course, one may recognize a granular appearance adjacent to a resolving cotton-wool spot,

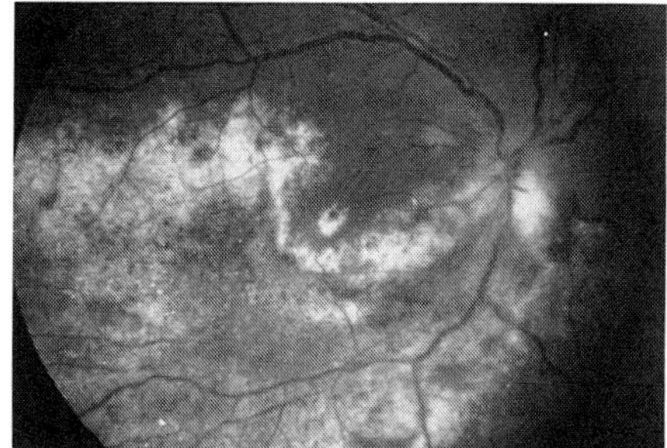

Figure 1 *Cytomegalovirus retinitis showing full-thickness granular retinal opacification with hard exudates and hemorrhages.*

sometimes with preretinal or intraretinal hemorrhages. This granular opacity increases in size and intensity over the ensuing weeks. CMV infection in the peripheral retina shows marked granularity, often with minimal or no retinal hemorrhages. As the infection spreads closer to the posterior pole, a more typical picture of a full-thickness retinitis with hard exudates and hemorrhages can be appreciated.

After successful anti–CMV retinitis treatment, the central portion of the infected retina is the first to show atrophic changes. What was before a full-thickness area of fluffy retinitis now becomes flatter and more granular, and the preretinal and intraretinal hemorrhages disappear (Fig 2). This atrophic granular appearance spreads from the central area of the opacity outward to the periphery. However, it is important to realize, in

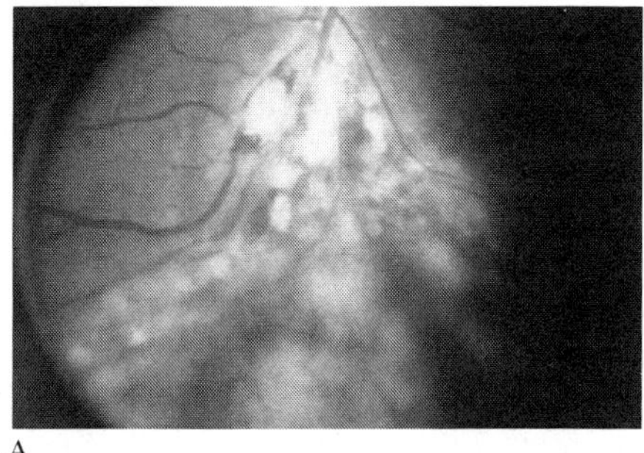

A

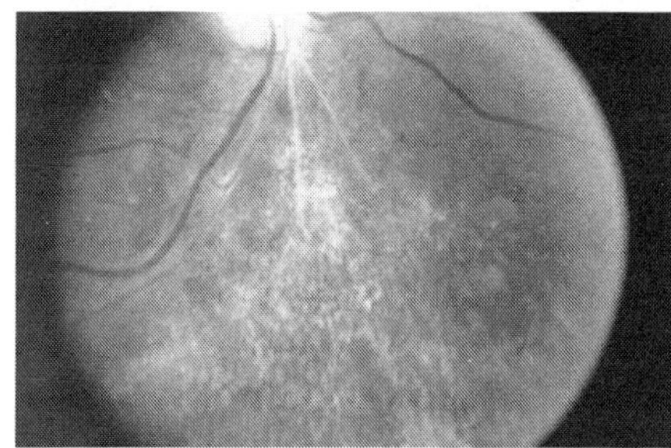

B

Figure 2 *Cytomegalovirus retinitis (A) before treatment and (B) 4 weeks after treatment.*

assessing treatment success, that the borders of the lesions and *not* the central area are indicative of continuing disease activity. Although there is a surprising lack of changes in the retinal pigment epithelium (RPE), the overlying retina does assume a moth-eaten atrophic appearance. In the chronic stages of the disease, large atrophic holes that may lead to retinal detachment are often seen. In recurrent disease, an area of seemingly atrophic retina at the border of the original CMV lesion becomes fluffy and opacified. Within weeks, preretinal and intraretinal hemorrhages are seen as the tail of active opacity gradually extends.

Treatment The issue of treatment in patients with CMV retinitis is difficult yet immediate, particularly in those patients who are relatively healthy and have only peripheral disease. Both ganciclovir and foscarnet are effective treatment modalities for CMV retinitis, with a response rate of 80 to 100% [10, 11, 18–29]. Moreover, treatment of CMV retinitis may prolong survival in AIDS patients. The median survival time has increased from 6 weeks in patients who receive no treatment, 1 month in those patients unresponsive to ganciclovir treatment, 3.1 months for those who respond partially, to 10 months in patients who respond completely to ganciclovir treatment [11]. Documentation of this increased survival time has prompted a more aggressive therapeutic approach in an attempt to preserve vision and prolong life. However, the side effects of both ganciclovir and foscarnet are severe [16].

Available Agents and Their Toxicities Only intravenous ganciclovir is approved for use in the United States. The initial, 2-week, high-dose induction therapy (5 mg/kg intravenously twice daily for 2 weeks) is begun to control infection and is followed by long-term maintenance therapy (5 mg/kg once every day, or 6 mg/kg once daily for 5 days each week), during which the ganciclovir is administered by an indwelling central venous catheter.

Ganciclovir's primary side effect is myelosuppression. Neutropenia, defined as an absolute neutrophil count of fewer than 500×10^6, has been reported to occur in 16 to 29% of patients treated with ganciclovir [11, 16]. This neutropenia is usually reversible but requires interruption of the drug therapy. Thrombocytopenia has been reported to occur in 5 to 10% of treated patients [14]. Moreover, zidovudine, used to treat AIDS, also has toxic effects on the bone marrow and therefore cannot be used at the full recommended dose (600 mg/day) concurrently with ganciclovir.

Like ganciclovir, foscarnet requires initial 2-week, high-dose induction therapy (60 mg/kg every 8 hours for 2 or 3 weeks) followed by long-term maintenance therapy (90 to 120 mg/kg/day 5 days weekly). Although foscarnet does not exert toxic effects on the bone marrow and, therefore, can be used concurrently with full-dose zidovudine, it is toxic to the kidneys. Renal dysfunction and metabolic abnormalities of calcium and magnesium have been reported in up to 30% of patients taking foscarnet [30–33]. Seizures have been reported in approximately 10% of patients receiving foscarnet [16].

Despite the impressive initial treatment response, active retinitis recurs in virtually all patients within 3 to 4 weeks after anti-CMV therapy is stopped [11–25]. Despite maintenance therapy, relapse has been reported in 18 to 50% of patients, though the time to relapse is much longer in patients on maintenance therapy than in untreated patients [11, 13, 16]. Most investigators believe that, given enough time, all patients on treatment will eventually relapse. Patients who relapse generally respond to a second course of induction therapy. If a patient relapses on one of the two therapeutic modalities, the other drug may be tried with some success. The resistance of CMV to foscarnet and ganciclovir has not been well studied.

Additional Complications of Therapy   An additional complication of anti-CMV treatment is that up to 29% of patients may develop retinal detachment during or after therapy [34]. Anti-CMV treatment may contribute to the development of retinal detachment by inhibiting scar formation [23–34]. However, Jabs and colleagues [11] found that a majority of their patients had retinal detachment at initial examination, before the institution of ganciclovir treatment. They also observed that all such patients had lesions extending anteriorly up to the pars plana. These investigators suggested that patients with lesions involving more than 50% of the retina have a greater rate of retinal detachment than do those with lesions involving less than 50% of the retina [11]. Irvine [35] has identified the presence of myopia as a risk factor for developing retinal detachments in patients with CMV retinitis. These retinal detachments are among the most difficult to repair because of extensive retinal necrosis and multiple (and often posterior) hole formation. Most investigators agree that these cases are not amenable to repair by scleral buckling alone [36]. The procedure of choice is pars plana vitrectomy with long-term silicone oil tamponade [37].

Recently, we studied 22 eyes of 19 AIDS patients who underwent pars plana vitrectomy and silicone oil injection after retinal detachment caused by CMV retinitis [38]. All patients but 1 were monitored until time of death. The median survival time postoperatively was 4 months, which was less than that for patients who respond completely to ganciclovir treatment but greater than that for patients who are partially responsive or unresponsive [11]. Only the duration of CMV retinitis, which may reflect immunological status, was predictive of survival. Anatomical reattachment with silicone oil occurred in 89.5% of our patients. However, the functional success was poor. Only 4 of 19 patients (21%) had better vision at the time of death than they had preoperatively; only 8 (42%) had vision of 5/200 or better at the time of death. A bimodal pattern of visual loss noted in these patients suggested that an intraoperative or immediately postoperative injury may have caused the early postoperative visual loss, whereas a continued postoperative retinitis or ischemia may have caused a later, more gradual, loss of vision. Only intraocular pressure (IOP) and optic nerve atrophy were found to predict visual outcome. We observed that the retinal vascular perfusion pressure in all eyes was low during operation, as evidenced by arteriolar pulsations with a low infusion pressure.

Pepose and associates [39] have documented retinal microvascular abnormalities, microaneurysms, and ischemic maculopathy in patients with AIDS; their ultrastructural studies showed occluded vessel lumina, swollen endothelial cells, thickened basal laminae, and degenerating pericytes. Using full-mount trypsin digest studies, we have demonstrated microvascular abnormalities consisting of an increased pericyte–to–endothelial cell ratio, ghost vessels, microaneurysms, and capillary dropout in patients with CMV retinitis [40]. We believe, therefore, that the early visual loss following repair of retinal detachment may be caused by intraoperative or immediate postoperative IOP increases and that the gradual loss in vision may be caused by a later increase in IOP, both instigating ischemia in an eye already compromised by microvasculopathy. This ischemia was evidenced by the development of optic nerve atrophy in 21 of 22 eyes (95.5%) that underwent repair of retinal detachment [38].

Relationship of Therapy to Prolonged Survival Although studies have shown that treatment of CMV retinitis prolongs survival, only the recent studies of ocular complications of AIDS have compared ganciclovir and foscarnet for the treatment of CMV retinitis in patients with AIDS in a randomized multicenter clinical trial. In October 1991, the treatment protocol for this study was suspended, owing to mortality differences between the two groups [41]: As of that date, 51% of patients who were assigned to the ganciclovir group had died, compared to 34% of patients assigned to the foscarnet group. Median survival time was 8.5 months for patients receiving ganciclovir compared to 12.6 months for patients receiving foscarnet. This excess mortality could not be explained fully by the differential antiretroviral drug use [16, 41]. Despite increased survival, there were no significant differences between the two groups in the rate of progression of retinitis.

The mechanism for prolonged survival after treatment of CMV retinitis is not known. We studied 412 cadaveric eyes from 206 autopsied AIDS patients and found 116 subjects (56%) had some organ infected with CMV. Of these 116 patients, 52 eyes of 33 patients had CMV retinitis diagnosed by histopathological examination. Of the 33 patients, 23 (70%) had received anti-CMV treatment and 10 (30%) had not. Patients treated for CMV retinitis had significantly fewer nonocular organs infected than did patients with untreated CMV retinitis ($p = .0005$). Moreover, patients treated for CMV retinitis had significantly fewer nonocular organs infected with CMV than did patients with untreated nonocular CMV infection ($p = .001$). Patients with untreated CMV retinitis were not statistically different from those with untreated nonocular CMV infection ($p = .37$) in terms of the number of organs infected with CMV. Of 32 patients with CMV retinitis diagnosed by histopathological examination, 7 of 9 (78%) untreated patients were found to have active disease, as compared to 5 of 23 (22%) treated patients. In 1 patient with CMV retinitis, the disease activity could not be determined.

The relationship between CMV infection of the optic nerve and the brain was also studied. Of 23 patients with CMV retinitis who had received treatment, 4 had optic nerve involvement. However, only 1 of these 4 had infection of the cerebrum. Of the 10 untreated patients with CMV retinitis, 2 had optic nerve involvement and 1 of these had CMV infection of the brain. In all cases of CMV infection involving the optic nerve, infection was limited to the prelaminar portion. We concluded that treatment of CMV retinitis reduces the number of CMV-infected nonocular organs and may also lessen the severity and control the spread of concurrent nonocular infection, both of which may prolong survival in AIDS patients. Moreover, we do not believe, based on this study, that CMV retinitis spreads to the brain via the optic nerve. Brain infection most likely occurs by the same mechanism as other systemic infections, namely by hematogenous dissemination [42, 43]. If our conclusion is correct, then the benefit of increased survival offered by systemic anti-CMV therapy would not be offered by local treatment modalities such as intraocular injections and sustained-release devices [44–46].

Current Research A topic of intense current research is the possibility of identifying patients at risk for developing CMV retinitis. Recent studies have indicated that CMV retinitis does not develop unless the CD4 lymphocyte counts are fewer than 50 cells/mm^3 [47, 48]. CMV retinitis may reflect severe immunosuppression that either results from or is a prerequisite for disseminated CMV infection. Recent evidence also suggests that an ischemic microvasculopathy, possibly caused by a direct HIV infection, may also predispose one to CMV retinitis [49].

We performed full-mount trypsin digest studies to determine the incidence of microvascular abnormalities in 30 eyes of 16 AIDS patients without CMV retinitis and in 20 eyes of 12 AIDS patients with CMV retinitis [49]. Microvascular abnormalities consisted of an increased pericyte–to–endothelial cell ratio, ghost vessels, microaneurysms, and capillary dropout. A pericyte–to–endothelial cell ratio of 5:1 or greater was found in 16 eyes (80%) with CMV retinitis and in 3 eyes (10%) without CMV retinitis. Three or more ghost vessels per high-power field were present in 14 eyes (70%) with CMV retinitis and in 3 eyes (10%) without CMV retinitis. We concluded that retinal microvascular abnormalities occurred to a greater degree in AIDS patients with CMV retinitis than in those without. These microvascular abnormalities were associated with immunosuppression as determined by the T-cell counts as well as the existence of systemic

CMV infection. We speculate that microvascular abnormalities, possibly as a reflection of generalized immunosuppression, may predispose AIDS patients to CMV retinitis.

Progressive Outer Retinal Necrosis

The acute retinal necrosis syndrome is characterized by an acute necrotizing retinitis with an associated moderate to severe hyalitis and anterior chamber reaction, classically occurring in otherwise healthy individuals [50–52]. A similar syndrome has been described in immunocompromised individuals, including patients with AIDS [53–55]. We reported 2 patients who were HIV-positive, both of whom developed a necrotizing retinitis associated with cutaneous herpes zoster infection [56]. Both patients had rapidly progressive disease and, despite intravenous acyclovir therapy, developed rhegmatogenous retinal detachments that were successfully repaired surgically. What distinguished our patients from those previously described was the primary involvement of the outer retina, with sparing of the inner retina as well as of the retinal vasculature until late in the disease process (Fig 3). Electron microscopy of the retinal biopsy specimen from 1 of the patients demonstrated viral particles consistent with the herpesvirus, and the polymerase chain reaction disclosed probable herpes zoster virus in the retinal biopsy specimen of the other patient. We believe this entity may represent a distinct form of acute retinal necrosis that is seen in AIDS patients [56]. Recently, Margolis and associates [57] described 5 AIDS patients with a similar presentation except that the retinitis began in the posterior pole, with little or no clinical evidence of vasculitis in 4 of the patients. The clinical and laboratory evidence suggested that varicella zoster virus was the causative agent in all 5 patients [57].

In its early stages, progressive outer retinal necrosis may be difficult to differentiate from peripheral CMV retinitis. However, its rapid progression in a circumferential pattern and sparing of the retinal vasculature will allow this disease to be more easily identified. Only 1 eye is usually affected in the initial presentation, but bilateral involvement is the rule, though the time to involvement of the second eye is highly variable, ranging from days to months in our experience. No adequate therapy currently exists, but ganciclovir appears to be more effective than acyclovir in stabilizing the infection [58].

Toxoplasma Retinochoroiditis

Toxoplasmosis is the most common AIDS-associated nonviral intracranial infection. However, ocular toxoplasmosis in patients with AIDS is relatively uncommon. Holland and associates [59] described 8 AIDS patients with toxoplasmal retinochoroiditis. They found no evidence that the disease originated in a preexisting chorioretinal scar. The lesions were

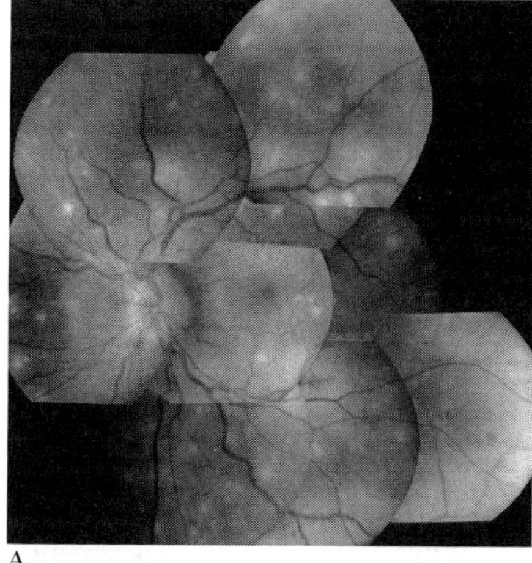

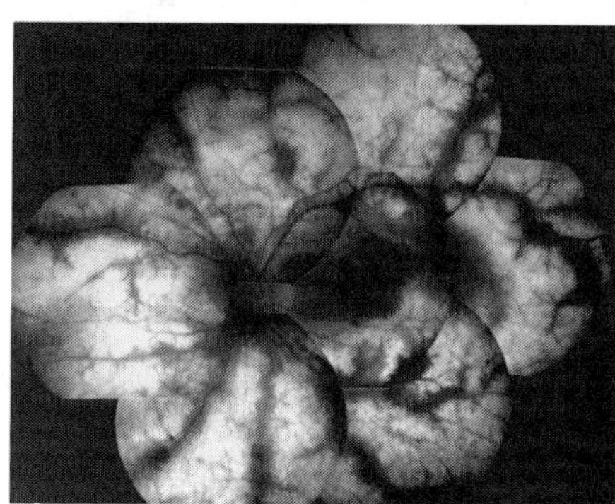

Figure 3 *Progressive outer retinal necrosis (A) on initial examination and (B) 6 days later. Established disease is distinguished by a primary involvement of the outer retina, with sparing of the inner retina as well as of the retinal vasculature.*

frequently bilateral and multifocal, and vitreous inflammation was a common clinical finding. The infections became clinically inactive with anti-*Toxoplasma* therapy (pyrimethamine, sulfadiazine, clindamycin, tetracycline, and spiramycin) but reactivated when therapy was stopped in 2 of 3 patients [59].

Holland and colleagues [59] emphasized that ocular toxoplasmosis in AIDS patients, unlike in immunocompetent patients, probably results from newly acquired infection. It is important to realize that ocular lesions can be the first manifestation of toxoplasmal infection in a number of AIDS patients with evidence of multisystem infection. Toxoplasmal retinochoroiditis can clinically mimic CMV retinitis and, similarly, toxoplasmal optic neuritis may be clinically indistinguishable from CMV optic neuritis [60]. Although the serological studies for toxoplasmosis may be helpful in distinguishing this disease, the test may be falsely negative owing to severe immunosuppression. Therefore, as with most other infections in AIDS, the diagnosis is mainly a clinical one. Usually AIDS patients with toxoplasmal retinitis show a moderate to severe degree of hyalitis; such vitreous inflammation is rarely seen in CMV retinitis.

Two important considerations are unique to the diagnosis and treatment of toxoplasmal retinochoroiditis in AIDS patients. First, a thorough systemic examination, especially for intracranial infection, must be done. Second, high-dose systemic steroids should not be a part of the treatment regimen, even if the toxoplasmal lesion is threatening the macula.

Syphilitic Chorioretinitis

The resurgence of ocular syphilis in patients with AIDS has recently been emphasized [61, 62]. Clinical presentations include uveitis, optic neuritis, and retinitis [63]. These patients may also exhibit dermatological and central nervous system manifestations. Gass and co-workers [62] described 6 patients with evidence of secondary syphilis who presented with characteristic findings that they have named *acute syphilitic posterior placoid chorioretinitis*. All 6 patients presented with hyalitis associated with bilateral large, solitary, placoid, pale yellowish subretinal lesions, usually showing evidence of central fading and a pattern of coarsely stippled hyperpigmentation of the RPE. Early-phase fluorescein angiography showed hypofluorescence in the area of the gray-white or yellow opacification and a stippled or leopard-spot pattern of nonfluorescence in the faded portion of the lesions. Late-phase angiograms showed staining at the level of the RPE that was most intense in the areas of gray-white or yellow change. There was evidence of shallow serous detachment of the overlying retina, peripheral chorioretinitis, mild papillitis, retinal perivasculitis, and iritis in a few eyes.

Tamesis and Foster [62] suggest that syphilis may pursue a more aggressive course in patients who are concurrently infected with HIV, rendering standard therapy for primary and secondary syphilis inadequate. These authors suggest that all patients with ocular syphilis be evaluated for HIV and vice versa. They currently admit all patients with ocular syphilis to the hospital and recommend an examination of the cerebrospinal fluid for cells, protein, and serological values. We treat all AIDS patients with ocular syphilis with the neurosyphilis treatment regimen of 12 to 24 MU/day of aqueous crystalline penicillin G intravenously for at least 10 days, followed by 2.4 MU/wk of benzathine penicillin G intramuscularly for 3 weeks.

Histoplasmosis

Disseminated histoplasmosis is a life-threatening infection in patients with AIDS. Recently, two reports have described ocular histoplasmosis in AIDS patients with the disseminated disease [64, 65]. Clinically, creamy white intraretinal and subretinal infiltrates that measure approximately 0.16 to 0.25 disc diameter in size were seen. Scattered intraretinal hemorrhage was also noted. All retinal infiltrates were found to have distinct borders. Although the clinical findings were nonspecific, the fact that the patients had disseminated histoplasmosis suggested the diagnosis of ocular histoplasmosis. On histopathological examination, the retina contained multiple white-tan lesions that measured up to 1 mm in diameter. Many were surrounded by a light tan halo. The lesions were located superficially and deep in the retina, and these retinal lesions contained *Histoplasma* organisms in all layers, sometimes with extension to subretinal and subhyaloid spaces. The lesions were often perivascular. The organisms were free or phagocytized within cells and were seen with or without infiltrative lymphocytes and histiocytes. Dispersion and intraretinal migration of the RPE with disruption of Bruch's membrane was seen adjacent to these retinal lesions. Intracytoplasmic yeast was seen in many RPE cells. Focal choroiditis, with histiocytes, lymphocytes, occasional plasma cells, and rare *Histoplasma* yeast, was observed near the retinitis. Owing to the potential devastating effect of this disease, ocular histoplasmosis must be considered in the differential diagnosis of any retinal choroiditis seen in an AIDS patient, particularly if the patient has lived in an area endemic for histoplasmosis.

Infectious Multifocal Choroiditis

The importance of multifocal choroiditis in AIDS patients was first emphasized by Rao and associates [66], who described 3 patients with *P. carinii* choroiditis. The choroidal circulation is one of the areas of highest blood flow in the body. In fact, more than 70% of all the blood in the globe at any one time can be found in the choriocapillaris [67]. In an experimental study, Stern and Ernest [68] demonstrated that injection of embolic microspheres into the lateral short posterior ciliary arteries resulted in delayed choroidal filling and multifocal necrosis of the RPE, with a concentration of the microspheres at the posterior pole. Yoneya and Tso [69] have found regional variations in the choriocapillaris's architectural pattern that account for increased choroidal flow to the macular region due to the presence of a more efficient lobular pattern. This lobular pattern in the posterior pole would also account for a multifocal distribution of lesions due to multiple embolic inclusions, be they microspheres or infectious emboli. Multifocal choroidal lesions from infectious causes are seen in patients with *P. carinii* pneumonia, disseminated *C. neoformans* infection, *M. avium-intracellulare* pneumonia, and other infections.

More than 80% of patients with AIDS develop *P. carinii* pneumonia and, in 60% of patients, it is the initial opportunistic infection [70]. Although initial treatment is generally effective, more than 60% of patients have a recurrence within 1 year unless they receive appropriate prophylaxis [71]. Aerosolized pentamidine is one such prophylactic agent, and it prevents recurrence in approximately 80% of patients for up to 1 year

[72]. Drug deposition, however, is limited to the lung, and there have been an increasing number of reports of extrapulmonary *P. carinii* infection [72, 73]. Presumably, extrapulmonary dissemination occurs during an early episode of *P. carinii* pneumonia, and then disease is reactivated at these sites after prophylaxis with aerosolized pentamidine [72, 73]. The eye may be one such site of reactivation.

The characteristic fundus changes of *P. carinii* choroiditis consist of slightly elevated, plaquelike, yellow-white lesions located in the choroid and unassociated with signs of intraocular inflammation (Fig 4) [66, 72]. By fluorescein angiography, these lesions tend to be hypofluorescent in the early phase and hyperfluorescent in the later phases (Fig 5) [72]. Although these patients may initially be asymptomatic or only minimally symptomatic, a thorough history of previous systemic infections must be undertaken. If disseminated *P. carinii* is suspected, an extensive examination including chest radiographs, arterial blood gas levels, liver function tests, and abdominal computed tomography must be done. Moreover, the patient must be hospitalized for a 3-week course of intravenous trimethoprim (20 mg/kg body weight/day) and sulfamethoxazole (100 mg/kg body weight/day) or pentamidine (4 mg/kg body weight/day). Within 3 to 12 weeks, most of the yellow-white lesions disappear, leaving no overlying pigmentary changes (Fig 6). The remaining lesions become smaller and develop sharper borders and slight granularity of overlying RPE. In all patients described in our initial reports, systemic dissemination of *P. carinii* choroiditis has been found [53, 72]. Subsequent studies have confirmed these findings [74, 75].

C. neoformans choroiditis in the presence of AIDS results in a multifocal pattern similar to that seen in *P. carinii* choroiditis [76; also Dugel and Rao, unpublished data]. We have recently examined 2 patients with multifocal choroiditis prior to the development of meningeal or systemic symptoms and signs. Both, however, did have nonspecific systemic complaints, including fever, chills, mild headache, malaise, and fatigue for several months. The visual complaints of intermittent blurred vision were equally nonspecific. Hematogenous spread most likely occurred weeks to months prior to

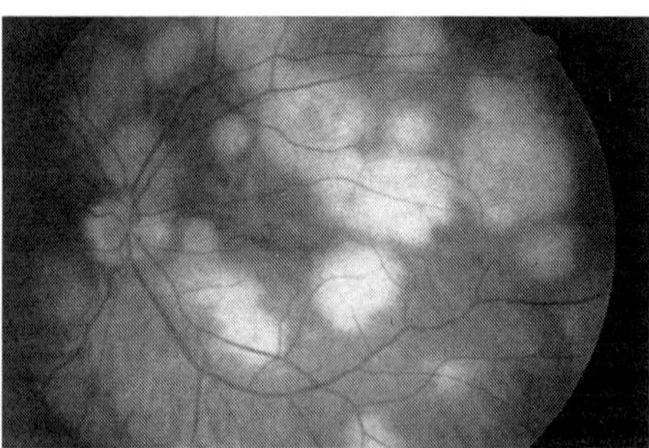

Figure 4 *Slightly elevated, plaquelike, yellow-white lesions, located in the choroid and unassociated with signs of intraocular inflammation, characterize the typical findings of* Pneumocystis carinii *choroiditis. (Reprinted with permission from [66].)*

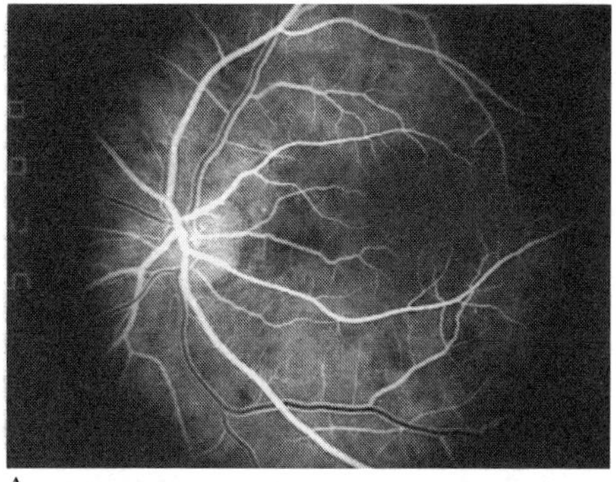

A

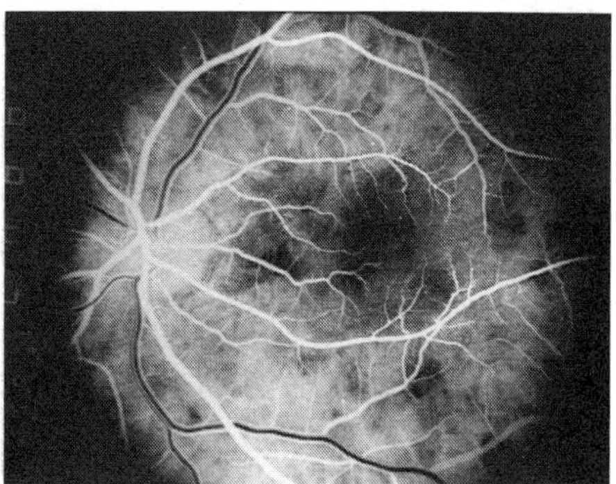

B

Figure 5 Pneumocystis carinii *choroiditis typically shows (A) early hypofluorescence and (B) late hyperfluorescence by fluorescein angiography. (Reprinted with permission from [72].)*

our examination, and thus it appears that intraocular involvement can occur without optic nerve extension of systemic infection. Ocular manifestations, then, may presage specific systemic manifestations of central nervous system disease, thereby leading to an early diagnosis of disseminated cryptococcosis. This multifocal pattern is nonetheless nonspecific, as such choroiditis is also seen in patients with *P. carinii, M. avium-intracellulare,* and *Mycobacterium kansasii* choroiditis [77].

In a recent study of 412 cadaveric eyes from 206 consecutive autopsied AIDS patients, we found 4 patients with bilateral *P. carinii* choroiditis [42, 43]. Each of these 4 patients showed disseminated lesions of *P. carinii* involving thoracic lymph nodes, spleen, and other viscera (Fig 7). Five patients had bilateral *C. neoformans* choroiditis, 2 had bilateral *M. avium-intracellulare* choroiditis, and 1 had *Histoplasma capsulatum* choroiditis. All patients with infectious choroiditis showed dissemination to visceral organs.

The choroid, perhaps more than any other part of the eye, demonstrates the importance of an ophthalmoscopic examination in AIDS patients. A multifocal choroiditis in an AIDS patient is an alarming, albeit a

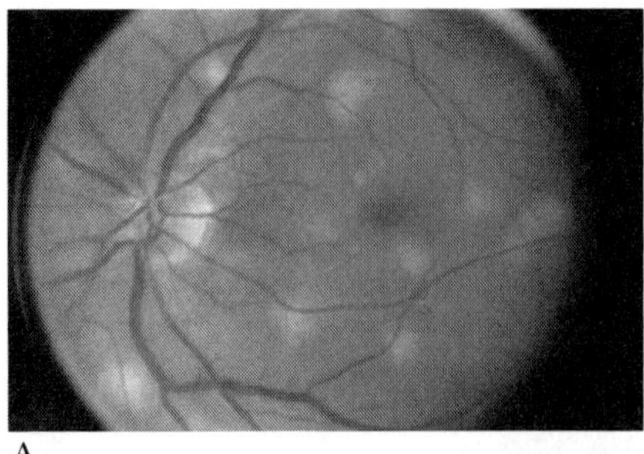

A

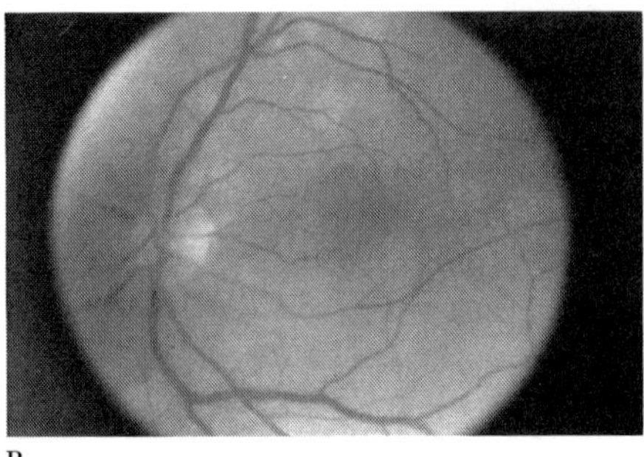

B

Figure 6 Pneumocystis carinii *choroiditis (A) on initial examination and (B) 3 months after treatment. (Reprinted with permission from [72].)*

nonspecific, sign. It is imperative that the ophthalmologist demand an exhaustive workup for disseminated infection in such a patient. Indeed, the ophthalmologist may have a lifesaving role in disease diagnosis and management of AIDS patients with multifocal choroiditis.

■ Anterior Segment Manifestations

Ocular Adnexal Kaposi's Sarcoma

Since the initial description of Kaposi's sarcoma in 1872 [78], two more aggressive variants of this tumor have been described. In 1959, an endemic variety was described in Africa, especially in Kenya and Nigeria, where it accounts for nearly 20% of all malignancies [79, 80]. The second variant, epidemic Kaposi's sarcoma, was first noted in renal transplant patients [81–84] and currently occurs in 30% of all patients with AIDS [85]. AIDS-associated Kaposi's sarcoma is particularly aggressive, disseminating to visceral organs (gastrointestinal tract, lung, and liver) in 20 to 50% of patients [86, 87].

Recent evidence suggests that AIDS-related Kaposi's sarcoma may have an infectious origin [88]. HIV in the pathogenesis of Kaposi's sarcoma has become evident from studies of transgenic mice bearing the HIV-1

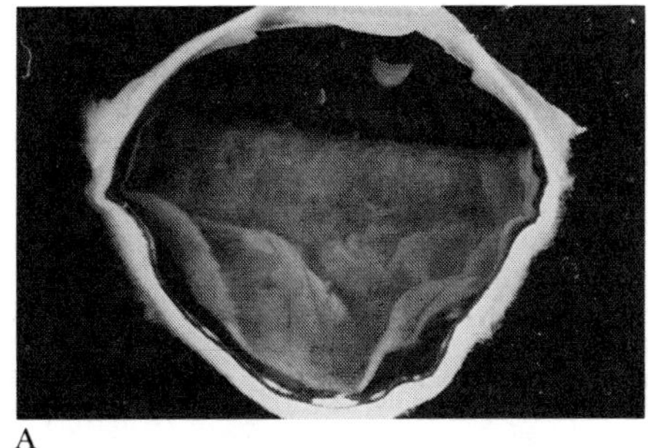

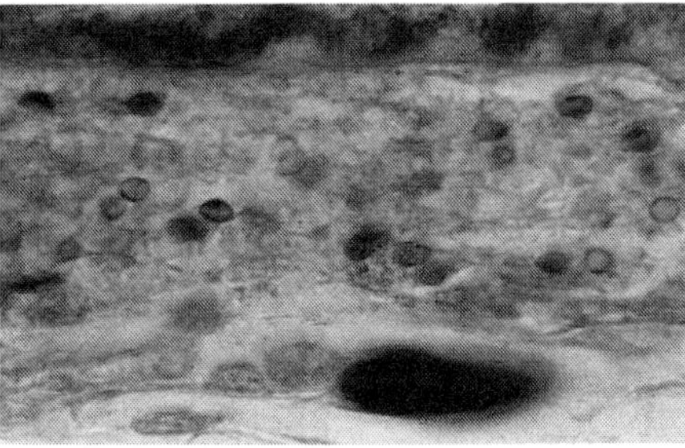

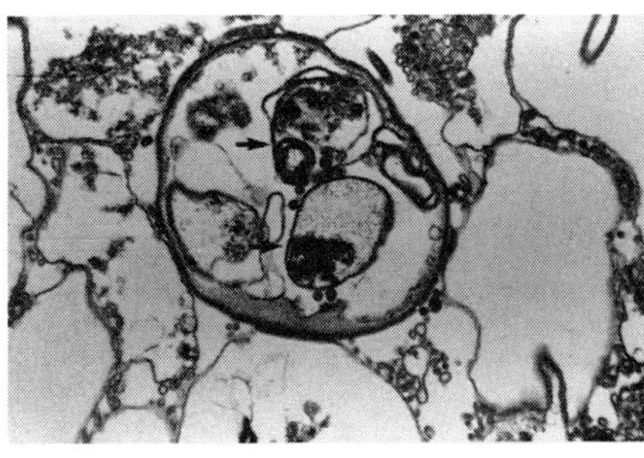

Figure 7 *(A) Gross examination of choroidal infiltrates due to* Pneumocystis carinii. *(B) Staining with Gomori's methenamine silver reveals* Pneumocystis *organisms within the choriocapillaris. (C) Electron microscopy shows typical organism containing multiple cysts.*

transactivator (TAT) gene under the control of the virus regulatory region (HIV-LTR) [89]. The HIV TAT protein has been shown to be a potent mitogen for human Kaposi's sarcoma–derived cell lines [90]. As in humans, these lesions in mice occur predominantly in the males, which suggests their development may be hormonally controlled.

Prior to 1981, ocular adnexal Kaposi's sarcoma had been reported in fewer than 25 patients, but today it occurs in approximately 20% of patients with AIDS-associated systemic Kaposi's sarcoma [91]. We have described three stages of ocular adnexal Kaposi's sarcoma in AIDS patients [92]. Clinically, stage I and stage II tumors are patchy and flat (less than

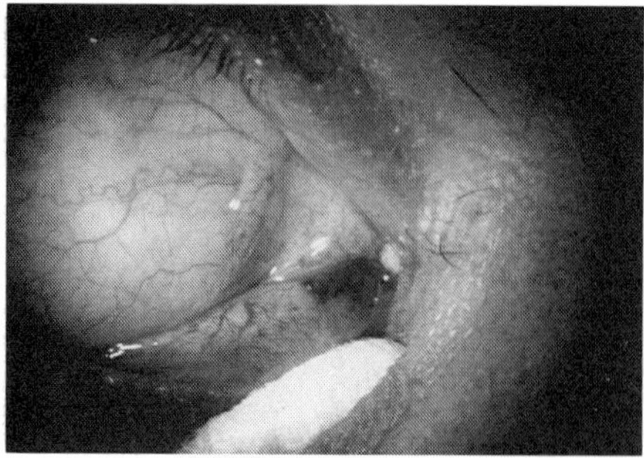

A

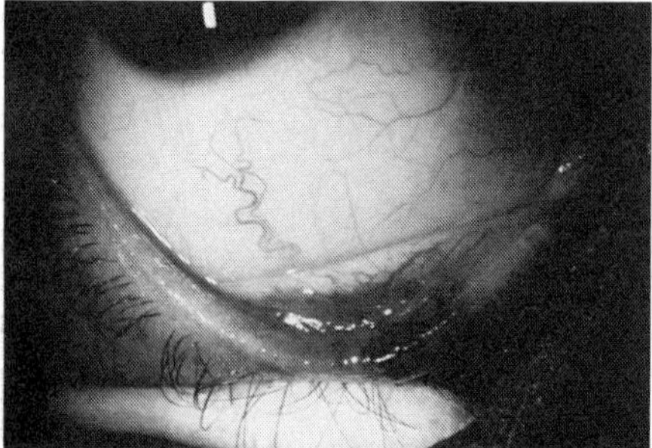

B

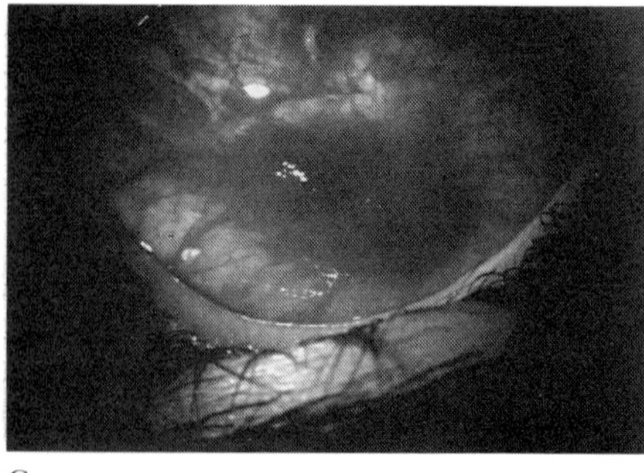

C

Figure 8 *Clinical stages of ocular adnexal Kaposi's sarcoma: (A) stage I, (B) stage II, and (C) stage III. (Reprinted with permission from [92].)*

3 mm in vertical height) and of less than 4 months' duration. Stage III tumors are nodular and elevated (greater than 3 mm in height) and of greater than 4 months' duration (Fig 8). Histologically, stage I tumor consists of thin dilated vascular channels lined by flat endothelial cells and often filled with erythrocytes. Mitotic figures are not usually seen. There is a moderate mononuclear cell infiltrate surrounding these abnormal vessels, but no spindle cells or split spaces are seen. Stage II lesions feature plump fusiform cells lining thin, dilated, empty vascular channels. Many

of these cells have a hyperchromatic nucleus. No mitotic cells are noted. A sparse inflammatory infiltrate composed of macrophages, plasma cells, and lymphocytes is seen. There are foci of immature spindle cells and early slit vessels. Stage III lesions are characterized by large aggregates of densely packed spindle cells with a hyperchromatic nucleus and an occasional mitotic figure. Between these spindle cells are slit spaces, many of which contain erythrocytes. Inflammatory cells are scanty (Fig 9). Based on the facts that recurrences are of an earlier stage than the primary tumor and all three stages can be present within the same lesion, we believe that these three stages are part of a continuum.

The increasing incidence of ocular manifestations of Kaposi's sarcoma has focused some attention recently on treatment. Radiotherapy is currently the treatment of choice [91], despite its significant expense and complications. Complications specifically reported after irradiation of ocular adnexal Kaposi's sarcoma include skin erythema [91], hair loss [91], and possible radiation-induced optic neuropathy [93]. Moreover, of 12 patients treated with radiotherapy for ocular adnexal Kaposi's sarcoma, the treatment was unsuccessful in 8 by 6 months (2 did not respond to treatment at all, 2 had recurrences after 4 months, and in 4 the tumors recurred after 6 months) [91].

Recently, we attempted to formulate a safer and more effective treatment regimen based on the clinical and histopathological stage of the tumor and its location [94]. Eighty-two patients with ocular adnexal Kaposi's sarcoma related to AIDS were examined, and 25 were selected to participate in this 3-year study. Of 14 patients with bulbar conjunctival Kaposi's sarcoma treated with surgical excision, 2 stage III tumors recurred during a follow-up that ranged from 8 to 31 months; no stage I or stage II lesion recurred. Of 7 patients with eyelid Kaposi's sarcoma treated with cryotherapy, 2 stage III tumors recurred during a follow-up period that ranged from 9 to 24 months; no stage I or stage II lesion recurred. Four patients with stage III Kaposi's sarcoma of the bulbar conjunctiva were treated with fluorescein angiography–based surgical excision. None of these lesions recurred during the follow-up that ranged from 4 to 8 months. We suggest that if treatment for ocular adnexal Kaposi's sarcoma in an AIDS patient is necessary for cosmetic reasons or to relieve functional difficulties, such as corneal irritation, recurrent corneal abrasions, tear film abnormalities, or obstruction of the visual axis, selection of the appropriate modalities should be based on tumor location and stage (whether by history and tumor height or by previous incisional biopsy). If the tumor is confined to the bulbar conjunctiva and is stage I or stage II, excisional biopsy with 1- to 2-mm tumor-free margins should be considered. Stage III Kaposi's sarcoma of the bulbar conjunctiva should be surgically excised, preferably after delineation by fluorescein angiography. Stage I and II Kaposi's sarcoma involving the eyelid may be treated with cryotherapy. However, stage III Kaposi's sarcoma of the eyelid may require radiotherapy. To avoid

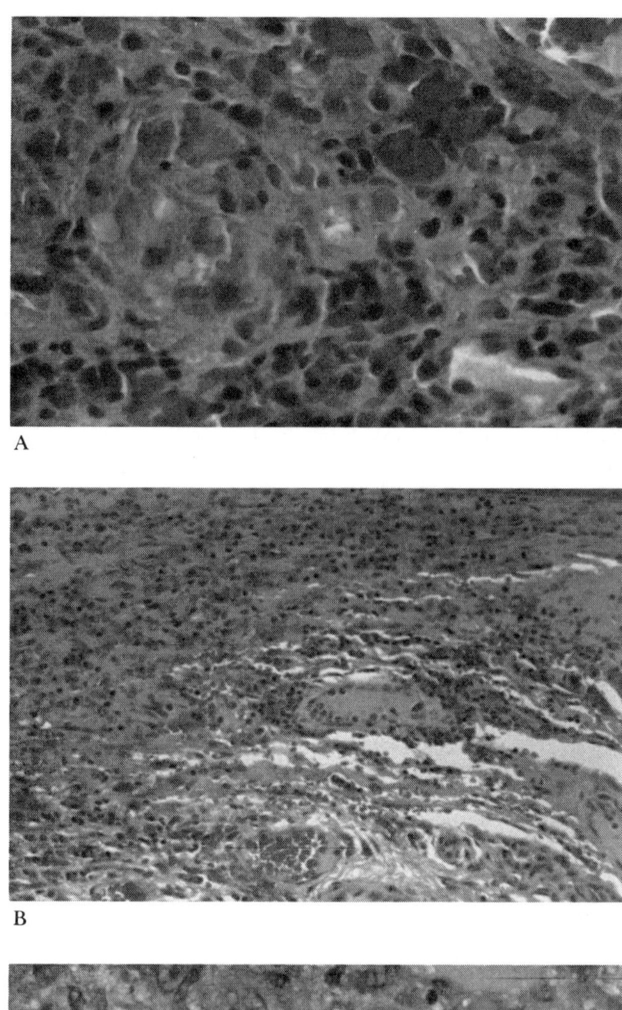
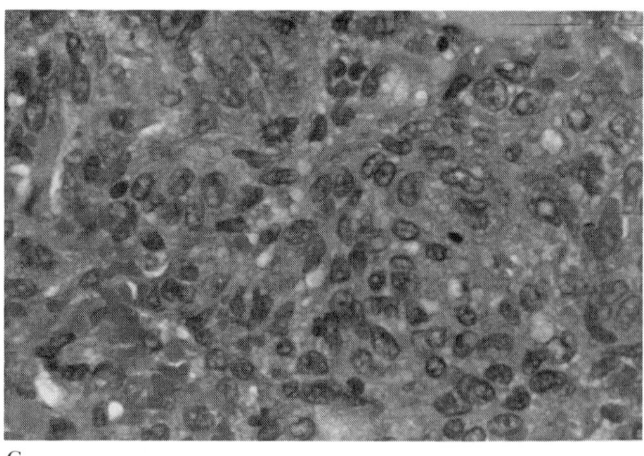

Figure 9 *Histological stages of ocular adnexal Kaposi's sarcoma: (A) stage I, (B) stage II, and (C) stage III. (Reprinted with permission from [92].)*

radiation-related complications, cryotherapy may be employed for such stage III lesions as long as the patient and practitioner understand that tumor recurrence is more likely and may necessitate repeat treatment [94]. It must be emphasized that when evaluating an AIDS patient with seemingly isolated ocular adnexal Kaposi's sarcoma, a full systemic examination for tumor dissemination must be performed. If chemotherapy is to be administered for systemic Kaposi's sarcoma, then the ophthalmologist should wait at least 4 to 6 weeks before treating the ocular adnexal lesions, as chemotherapy may reduce the tumor size to a point where it is no longer problematic.

Molluscum Contagiosum

Molluscum contagiosum lesions shed viral particles in the conjunctival cul-de-sac, causing a follicular conjunctivitis that persists until the eyelid margin lesion spontaneously heals or is excised. The lesions are usually 2 to 3 mm in diameter and typically have an unbilicated center. In healthy individuals, they are usually unilateral. In AIDS patients, we have noted a tendency for these lesions to be multiple and bilateral. The molluscum virus is a DNA virus belonging to the poxvirus family. If AIDS patients have significant functional difficulties, such as a persistent conjunctivitis, we surgically excise these lesions with cautery or cryotherapy to the base.

Herpes Zoster Ophthalmicus

Apparently young healthy individuals who present with herpes zoster lesions of the face or eyelids should be suspected of having AIDS and should be tested for HIV. We have examined approximately 20 young, homosexual men presenting with herpes zoster lesions of face and eyelids, all of whom tested positively for HIV [7]. Corneal involvement may cause a persistent, chronic keratitis [95]. Treatment consists of intravenous (1.5 mg/mm^2/day for 7 to 10 days) and topical acyclovir (5% ointment).

Microvascular Conjunctival Changes

A recent study showed bilateral presence of dilated, short segments of conjunctival vessels in 75% of patients with AIDS or AIDS-related conditions [96]. Hemorrheological abnormalities, such as increased red blood cell aggregation, high fibrinogen levels, and above-normal levels of plasma viscosity and quantitative IgG, were noted in most HIV-positive patients. The investigators postulated that these hemorrheological abnormalities may contribute to vascular damage and ocular ischemic lesions in the retina (cotton-wool spots) and conjunctiva (dilated vessels) of these patients. As in Kaposi's sarcoma, the possibility exists that this is an infectious microvasculopathy, perhaps due to HIV.

Keratitis

AIDS does not appear to predispose individuals to bacterial keratitis but, once established, these keratic infections are severe and more likely to cause perforation [7]. Fungal keratitis can occur in patients with AIDS without any history of trauma, topical steroid use, or blepharitis. Herpes simplex keratitis does not appear to occur with higher frequency in patients with AIDS but, when it does occur, tends to take a prolonged course and have a limbal predisposition [7]. Recently, a coarse superficial punctate keratitis with a minimal conjunctival reaction has been reported in patients with AIDS [97]. Electron microscopy of the epithelial scrapings revealed an obligate, intracellular, protozoal parasite from the Microsporidia family to be responsible for this atypical keratitis.

Infectious Conjunctival Granuloma

Recently, a solitary granulomatous conjunctivitis has been reported as an initial manifestation of cryptococcal infection, preceding HIV seroconversion by more than 1 month [98]. A 36-year-old woman with a 1-month history of temporal conjunctival hyperemia and a painful, progressive enlarging mass in her right eye was referred to the authors [98]. She had been treated with topical antibiotics and corticosteroids, which alleviated her symptoms slightly. A diagnostic biopsy of the granuloma disclosed connective tissue that was infiltrated with lymphocytes, plasma cells, and segmented granulocytes. The granulocytes were interspersed with organisms resembling yeast that were arranged singularly or in irregular groups. Immunofluorescent staining was consistent with a diagnosis of *C. neoformans*, which was confirmed by additional cultures and a positive serological antigen test. One month after the initial diagnosis was made, Western blot analysis demonstrated HIV seroconversion. The authors presumed a local ocular infection, although metastatic spread could not be ruled out as a bronchial lavage was not performed [98]. We believe that the differential diagnosis of a conjunctival granuloma in an AIDS patient should include sarcoidosis, tuberculosis, and mycotic infection. As with all other infections in AIDS, the possibility of dissemination must be entertained and aggressively sought.

■ Conclusion

The pathogenesis of ocular infections in AIDS patients is not known. To consider these varied infections simply opportunistic would be, at best, inadequate. It has become clear that so-called opportunistic infections (such as fungal chorioretinitis) seen in other forms of immunosuppression (such as congenital immune defects and chemical- or radiation-induced immunosuppression) are not seen in AIDS patients. On the other hand, infections such as *P. carinii* choroiditis have thus far been described primarily in AIDS patients and not in patients with other forms of immunosuppression. It is, therefore, intriguing to speculate that HIV may play an active role in promoting or perhaps selecting certain types of infections. Indeed, there is evidence for the active role of HIV in initiating Kaposi's sarcoma [88–90] and CMV retinitis [99]. Thus, many of the infections described herein may not be opportunistic at all, and the avoidance of this term may eventually lead to a better understanding of the pathogenic mechanism of infections in AIDS patients.

The role of the ophthalmologist in the diagnosis of disease and management of AIDS patients is becoming increasingly important. Not only does the eye reflect systemic disease, but often ocular symptoms may precede systemic manifestations. In the AIDS patient, the ophthalmologist can make not only a sight-saving but also a lifesaving diagnosis. Hence, it is the ophthalmologist's responsibility to provide a thorough and accurate ophthalmological examination as well as a careful and pertinent systemic evaluation, timely referrals, and periodic follow-up care.

This work was supported in part by core grant EYO3040 from the National Eye Institute, National Institutes of Health, Bethesda, MD, and by Research to Prevent Blindness, Inc., New York, NY. Dr. Rao is a recipient of the Dolly Green Scholar Award from Research to Prevent Blindness, Inc. Dr. Dugel is a recipient of the 1992–1993 Heed Ophthalmic Foundation Award.

■ References

1. Centers for Disease Control. HIV/AIDS surveillance report. Atlanta: CDC, December 1990:1
2. Centers for Disease Control. Update. Acquired immunodeficiency syndrome—United States, 1989. MMWR 1990;39:81
3. Ortiz R, Aaberg TM. Human immunodeficiency virus—disease epidemiology and nosocomial infection. Am J Ophthalmol 1991;112:35
4. DeGruttola V, Fineberg HV. Estimating prevalence of HIV infection. Considerations in the design and analysis of a national seroprevalence survey. J Acquir Immune Defic Syndr 1989;2:472
5. Fleming DW, Cochi SL, Steece RS, Hull HF. Acquired immunodeficiency syndrome in low-incidence areas. How safe is unsafe sex? JAMA 1987;258:785
6. Centers for Disease Control. Human immunodeficiency virus infection in the United States. A review of current knowledge. MMWR 1987;36:1
7. Frangieh GT, Dugel PU, Rao NA. Ocular manifestations of acquired immunodeficiency syndrome. Curr Opin Ophthalmol 1992;3:228
8. Holland GN, Pepose JS, Pettit TH, et al. Acquired immunodeficiency syndrome: ocular manifestations. Ophthalmology 1983;90:859
9. Palestine AG, Rodrigues MM, Maches AM, et al. Ophthalmic involvement in acquired immunodeficiency syndrome. Ophthalmology 1984;91:1092

10. Schuman JS, Orellana J, Friedman AH, Teich SA. Acquired immunodeficiency syndrome (AIDS). Surv Ophthalmol 1987;31:384
11. Jabs DA, Enger C, Bartlett JG. Cytomegalovirus retinitis and acquired immunodeficiency syndrome. Arch Ophthalmol 1989;107:75
12. Jabs DA, Green WR, Fox R, et al. Ocular manifestations of acquired immune deficiency syndrome. Ophthalmology 1989;96:1092
13. Gross JG, Bozzette SA, Mathews WC, et al. Longitudinal study of cytomegalovirus retinitis in acquired immune deficiency syndrome. Ophthalmology 1990;97:681
14. Holland GN, Sison RF, Jatulis DE, et al. The UCLA CMV Retinopathy Study Group: survival of patients with the acquired immune deficiency syndrome after development of cytomegalovirus retinopathy. Ophthalmology 1990;97:204
15. Centers for Disease Control. HIV prevalence estimates in AIDS case projections for United States: report based upon a workshop. MMWR 1990;39(suppl):15
16. Jabs DA. Treatment of cytomegalovirus retinitis—1992. Arch Ophthalmol 1992;110:185
17. Pepose JS. Cytomegalovirus infections of the retina. In: Ryan SJ, ed. Retina, vol 2. St Louis: Mosby, 1989
18. Felsenstein D, D'Amico DJ, Hirsch MS, et al. Treatment of cytomegalovirus retinitis with 9-[2-hydroxy-1-(hydroxymethyl) ethoxymethyl] guanine. Ann Intern Med 1985;103:377
19. Palestine AG, Stevens G Jr, Lane HC, et al. Treatment of cytomegalovirus retinitis with dihydroxy propoxymethyl guanine. Am J Ophthalmol 1986;101:95
20. Collaborative DHPG Treatment Study Group. Treatment of serious cytomegalovirus infections with 9-(1,3-dihydroxy-2-propoxymethyl) guanine in patients with AIDS and other immunodeficiencies. N Engl J Med 1986;314:801
21. Rosecan LR, Stahl-Bayliss CM, Kalman CM, Laskin OL. Antiviral therapy for cytomegalovirus retinitis in AIDS with dihydroxy propoxymethyl guanine. Am J Ophthalmol 1986;101:405
22. Jabs DA, Wingard JR, de Bustros S, et al. BW B759U for cytomegalovirus retinitis. Intraocular drug penetration. Arch Ophthalmol 1986;104:1436
23. Holland GN, Sakamoto MJ, Hardy D, et al. Treatment of cytomegalovirus retinopathy in patients with acquired immunodeficiency syndrome. Use of the experimental drug 9-[2-hydroxy-1-(hydroxymethyl) ethoxymethyl] guanine. Arch Ophthalmol 1986;104:794
24. D'Amico DJ, Talamo JH, Felenstein D, et al. Ophthalmoscopic and histologic findings in cytomegalovirus retinitis treated with BW-B759U. Arch Ophthalmol 1986;104:1788
25. Henderly DE, Freeman WR, Causey DM, Rao NA. Cytomegalovirus retinitis and response to therapy with ganciclovir. Ophthalmology 1987;94:425
26. Holland GN, Sidikaro Y, Kreiger AE, et al. Treatment of cytomegalovirus retinopathy with ganciclovir. Ophthalmology 1987;94:815
27. Jabs DA, Newman C, de Bustros S, Polk BF. Treatment of cytomegalovirus retinitis with ganciclovir. Ophthalmology 1987;94:824
28. Orellana J, Teich SA, Friedman AH, et al. Combined short- and long-term therapy for the treatment of cytomegalovirus retinitis using ganciclovir (BW B759U). Ophthalmology 1987;94:8311
29. Lastrin OL, Cederberg DM, Mills J, et al. Ganciclovir for the treatment and suppression of serious infections caused by cytomegalovirus. Am J Med 1987;83:201
30. Walinsley SL, Chew E, Read SE, et al. Treatment of cytomegalovirus retinitis with trisodium phosphonoformate hexahydrated (foscarnet). J Infect Dis 1988;157:569
31. LeHoang P, Girard B, Robinet M, et al. Foscarnet in the treatment of cytomegalovirus retinitis in the acquired immune deficiency syndrome. Ophthalmology 1989;96:865

32. Jacobson MA, O'Donnell JJ, Mills J. Foscarnet treatment of cytomegalovirus retinitis in patients with acquired immunodeficiency syndrome. Antimicrob Agents Chemother 1989;33:736

33. Palestine AG, Polis MA, deSmet MD, et al. A randomized, controlled trial of foscarnet in the treatment of cytomegalovirus retinitis in patients with AIDS. Ann Intern Med 1991;115:665

34. Freeman WR, Henderly DE, Wan WL, et al. Prevalence, pathophysiology, and treatment of rhegmatogenous retinal detachment in treated cytomegalovirus retinitis. Am J Ophthalmol 1987;103:527

35. Irvine AR. Treatment of rhegmatogenous retinal detachment in AIDS patients with cytomegalovirus retinitis. Trans Am Ophthalmol Soc 1991;LXXXIX:349

36. Holland GN. The management of retinal detachments in patients with acquired immunodeficiency syndrome. Arch Ophthalmol 1991;109:791

37. Sidikaro Y, Silver L, Holland GN, Krieger A. Rhegmatogenous retinal detachments in patients with AIDS and necrotizing retinal infections. Ophthalmology 1991;98:129

38. Dugel PU, Liggett PE, Lee MB, et al. Repair of retinal detachment caused by cytomegalovirus retinitis in patients with the acquired immunodeficiency syndrome. Am J Ophthalmol 1991;112:235

39. Pepose JS, Holland GN, Nestor MS, et al. Acquired immune deficiency syndrome. Pathogenic mechanisms of ocular disease. Ophthalmology 1985;92:4772

40. Rao K, Dugel PU, Morinelli EN, Rao N. Retinal microvascular abnormalities in the acquired immunodeficiency syndrome. Invest Ophthalmol 1992;33:742

41. Studies of Ocular Complications of AIDS Research Group in Collaboration with the AIDS Clinical Trials Group. Mortality in patients with acquired immunodeficiency syndrome treated with either foscarnet or ganciclovir for cytomegalovirus retinitis. N Engl J Med 1992;326:213

42. Morinelli EN, Dugel PU, Rao NA. Infectious multifocal choroiditis and systemic dissemination in AIDS patients. Presented at the American Academy of Ophthalmology, Annual Meeting, Nov 8–12, 1992

43. Morinelli EN, Dugel PU, Rao NA. Opportunistic intraocular infection and its systemic association in AIDS patients. Trans Am Ophthalmol Soc (in press)

44. Henry K, Cantrill HL, Fletcher C, et al. Use of intravitreal ganciclovir (dihydroxy propoxymethyl guanine) for cytomegalovirus retinitis in a patient with AIDS. Am J Ophthalmol 1987;103:17

45. Cochereau-Massin I, LeHoang P, Lautier-Fran M, et al. Efficacy and tolerance of intravitreal ganciclovir in cytomegalovirus retinitis in the acquired immune deficiency syndrome. Ophthalmology 1991;98:1348

46. Sanborn GE, Araud R, Torti RE, et al. Sustained-release ganciclovir therapy for treatment of cytomegalovirus retinitis. Arch Ophthalmol 1992;110:188

47. Hochster H, Dieterich D, Bozzette S, et al. Toxicity of combined ganciclovir and zidovudine for cytomegalovirus disease associated with AIDS. An AIDS clinical trial group study. Ann Intern Med 1990;113:111

48. Kuppermann BD, Petty JG, Richman DD, et al. Cross sectional prevalence of CMV retinitis in AIDS patients: correlation with CD4 counts. Invest Ophthalmol Vis Sci 1992;33:750

49. Rao K, Dugel PU, Morinelli EN, Rao NA. Retinal microvascular abnormalities in the acquired immunodeficiency syndrome. Invest Ophthalmol Vis Sci 1992;33:742

50. Urayama A, Yamada N, Sasaki T, et al. Unilateral acute uveitis with retinal periarteritis and detachment. Jpn J Clin Ophthalmol 1971;25:607

51. Fischer JP, Lewis ML, Blumenkranz M, et al. The acute retinal necrosis syndrome. Part 1. Clinical manifestations. Ophthalmology 1971;25:607

52. Culbertson WW, Blumenkranz MS, Hines H, et al. The acute retinal necrosis syndrome. Part 2. Histopathology and etiology. Ophthalmology 1982;89:1317

53. Freeman WR, Thomas EL, Rao NA, et al. Demonstration of herpes group virus in acute retinal necrosis syndrome. Am J Ophthalmol 1986;102:701

54. Jabs DA, Schachat AP, Liss R, et al. Presumed varicella zoster retinitis in immunocompromised patients. Retina 1987;7:9

55. Chess J, Marcus DM. Zoster-related bilateral retinal necrosis syndrome as a presenting sign in AIDS. Ann Ophthalmol 1988;20:431

56. Forster DJ, Dugel PU, Frangieh GT, et al. Rapidly progressive outer retinal necrosis in the acquired immunodeficiency syndrome. Am J Ophthalmol 1990;110:341

57. Margolis TP, Lowder CY, Holland GN, et al. Varicella-zoster virus retinitis in patients with the acquired immunodeficiency syndrome. Am J Ophthalmol 1991;112:119

58. Forster DJ, Dugel PU, Frangieh GT, et al. Rapidly progressive outer retinal necrosis in the acquired immunodeficiency syndrome [letter]. Am J Ophthalmol 1991;111:256

59. Holland GN, Engstrom RE, Glasgow BJ, et al. Ocular toxoplasmosis in patients with the acquired immunodeficiency syndrome. Am J Ophthalmol 1988;106:653

60. Grossniklaus HE, Specht CS, Allaire G, Lewitt JA. *Toxoplasma gondii* retinochoroiditis and optic neuritis in AIDS. Ophthalmology 1990;97:1342

61. Gass JDM, Braunstein RA, Chenoweth RG. Acute syphilitic posterior placoid chorioretinitis. Ophthalmology 1990;97:1288–1297

62. Tamesis RR, Foster CS. Ocular syphilis. Ophthalmology 1990;97:1281–1287

63. Passo MS, Rosenbaum JT. Ocular syphilis in patients with human immunodeficiency virus infection. Am J Ophthalmol 1988;106:1–6

64. Specht SC, Mitchell KT, Bauman AE, Gupta M. Ocular histoplasmosis with retinitis in a patient with acquired immunodeficiency syndrome. Ophthalmology 1991;98:1356–1359

65. Macher A, Rodrigues MN, Kaplan W, et al. Disseminated bilateral chorioretinitis due to *Histoplasma capsulatum* in a patient with the acquired immunodeficiency syndrome. Ophthalmology 1985;92:1159–1164

66. Rao NA, Zimmerman PL, Boyer D, et al. A clinical, histopathologic and electron microscopic study of *Pneumocystis carinii* choroiditis. Am J Ophthalmol 1989;107:218

67. Parver LM, Anker T, Carpenter DO. Choroidal blood flow as a heat dissipating mechanism in the macula. Am J Ophthalmol 1980;89:641

68. Stern WH, Ernest JT. Microsphere occlusion of the choriocapillaris in rhesus monkeys. Am J Ophthalmol 1974;78:438

69. Yoneya S, Tso MOM. Angioarchitecture of the human choroid. Arch Ophthalmol 1987;105:681

70. Suffredini AF, Mansur H. *Pneumocystis carinii* infection in AIDS. In: Wormser GP, Stahl RE, Bottone EJ, eds. Acquired immune deficiency syndrome and other manifestations of HIV infection. Park Ridge, NJ: Noyes Publications, 1987:445–477

71. Centers for Disease Control. Guidelines for prophylaxis against *Pneumocystis carinii* pneumonia for persons infected with human immunodeficiency virus. MMWR 1989;38:1

72. Dugel PU, Rao NA, Forster DJ, et al. *Pneumocystis carinii* choroiditis after long-term aerosolized pentamidine therapy. Am J Ophthalmol 1990;110:113

73. Dugel PU, Rao NA, Forster DJ, et al. *Pneumocystis carinii* choroiditis after long-term aerosolized pentamidine therapy [letter]. Am J Ophthalmol 1991;111:118

74. Rosenblatt MA, Cunningham C, Friedman AH. Choroidal lesions in patients with AIDS. Br J Ophthalmol 1990;744:610

75. Koser MW, Jampol LM, MacDonnel K. Treatment of *Pneumocystis carinii* choroidopathy. Arch Ophthalmol 1990;108:1214

76. Carney MD, Combs JL, Waschler W. Cryptococcal choroiditis. Retina 1990;10:27
77. Dugel PU, Foster DJ, Rao NA. Opportunistic choroiditis in AIDS. Presented at the American Academy of Ophthalmology, Annual Meeting, Anaheim, CA, Oct 13–17, 1991
78. Kaposi M. Idiopathisches multiple pigmentsarkom der haut. Arch Dermatol Syphilib 1872;4:265
79. Taylor JF, Templeton AC, Vogel CL, et al. Kaposi's sarcoma in Uganda: a clinico-pathological study. Int J Cancer 1971;8:122
80. Templeton AC, Hull MSR. Distribution of tumours in Uganda. Recent Results Cancer Res 1973;41:1
81. Penn I. Kaposi's sarcoma in organ transplant recipients: report of 20 cases. Transplantation 1979;27:8
82. Klepp O, Dahl O, Stenwig JT. Association of Kaposi's sarcoma and prior immuno-suppressive therapy. Cancer 1978;42:2626
83. Harwood AR, Osoba D, Hofstader SL, et al. Kaposi's sarcoma in recipients of renal transplants. Am J Med 1979;67:759
84. Gange RW, Jones EW. Kaposi's sarcoma and immunosuppressive therapy: an appraisal. Clin Exp Dermatol 1978;3:135
85. Haimkos HW, Drotman DP, Morgan M. Prevalence of Kaposi's sarcoma among patients with AIDS [letter]. N Engl J Med 1985;312:1518
86. Friedman-Kien AE, Laubenstein LJ, Rubinstein P, et al. Disseminated Kaposi's sarcoma in homosexual men. Ann Intern Med 1982;96:693
87. Muggia FM, Lonberg M. Kaposi's sarcoma and AIDS. Med Clin North Am 1986;70:139
88. Dugel PU, Gill PS, Frangieh GT, et al. Particles resembling retrovirus and conjunctival Kaposi's sarcoma. Am J Ophthalmol 1990;110:86
89. Vogel J, Hinrichs SH, Reynolds PA, et al. The HIV "tat" gene induces dermal lesions resembling Kaposi's sarcoma in transgenic mice. Nature 1988;335:606
90. Ensoli B, Nakamura S, Salahuddin SZ, et al. AIDS Kaposi's sarcoma cells express cytokines with autocrine and paracrine growth effects. Science 1989;243:223
91. Shuler JD, Holland GN, Miles SA, et al. Kaposi's sarcoma of the conjunctiva and eyelids associated with the acquired immunodeficiency syndrome. Arch Ophthalmol 1989;107:858
92. Dugel PU, Gill PS, Frangieh GT, Rao NA. Ocular adnexal Kaposi's sarcoma in acquired immunodeficiency syndrome. Am J Ophthalmol 1990;110:500
93. Howard GM, Jakobiec FA, DeVoe AG. Kaposi's sarcoma of the conjunctiva. Am J Ophthalmol 1975;79:420
94. Dugel PU, Gill PS, Frangieh GT, Rao NA. Treatment of ocular adnexal Kaposi's sarcoma in the acquired immunodeficiency syndrome. Ophthalmology 1992;29:1127
95. Engstrom RE, Holland GN. Chronic herpes zoster virus associated with the acquired immunodeficiency syndrome. Am J Ophthalmol 1988;105:556
96. Engstrom RE, Holland GN, Hardy DW, Meisselman HJ. Hemorrheologic abnormalities in patients with human immunodeficiency virus infection and ophthalmic microvasculopathy. Am J Ophthalmol 1990;109:153
97. Pepose JS. Patient with AIDS presents with keratoconjunctivitis. Arch Ophthalmol 1990;108:1224
98. Balmes R, Bialasiewicz AA, Busse H. Conjunctival cryptococcosis preceding human immunodeficiency virus seroconversion. Am J Ophthalmol 1992;113:7719
99. Skoluik PR, Pomerantz RI, de la Monte SM, et al. Dual infection of retina with human immunodeficiency virus type I and cytomegalovirus. Am J Ophthalmol 1989;107:361

Acute Retinal Necrosis and Similar Retinitis Syndromes

William W. Culbertson, M.D.

Sally S. Atherton, Ph.D.

■ Acute Retinal Necrosis

Although acute retinal necrosis (ARN) syndrome is often considered a newly recognized disease, it has, in fact, been 20 years since it was first described in the Japanese literature by Urayama and associates [1]. This disease was known at the time as *Kirisawa uveitis,* named after Professor Nagonori Kirisawa. In this early report, Urayama described 6 patients with unilateral acute uveitis and retinal periarteritis and detachment. The distinguishing features of the syndrome—peripheral retinal necrosis, retinal arteritis, vitritis, and late rhegmatogenous retinal detachment— ineffective treatment, and a poor visual prognosis were emphasized. Five years later, cases began to be reported in the West by authors who were apparently unaware of this original report. Young and Bird [2], in London in 1978, reported 4 healthy patients with bilateral peripheral necrotizing retinitis, which they called *bilateral acute retinal necrosis,* or BARN. Since then, it has become apparent that many cases are unilateral, and the term *acute retinal necrosis* has become the most commonly used name for this syndrome worldwide.

ARN is a disorder of varying severity manifested by acute, primarily peripheral necrotizing retinitis, vitritis, retinal arteritis, occasional optic neuropathy, and late rhegmatogenous retinal detachment. ARN appears to represent one specific expression of a spectrum of diseases that have in common acute retinitis caused by a herpesvirus, either varicella zoster (VZV) or herpes simplex virus (HSV). We can group these disorders under the inclusive title of *acute herpesvirus retinitis.*

In addition to ARN, rapidly progressive outer retinal necrosis, which occurs in the acquired immunodeficiency syndrome (AIDS), and a diffuse fulminant herpetic retinitis may be identified as syndromes caused by herpesviruses that are clinically distinct from ARN but that share some similar features. These three syndromes differ from one another in terms of the patient's immune and inflammatory response to the virus.

Clinical Features

ARN syndrome typically begins with anterior granulomatous uveitis, with episcleral injection, granulomatous keratic precipitates, elevated pressure, and ocular pain, especially on eye movement. Within a day or two, there are usually posterior segment findings including posterior, focal, deep retinal thumbprintlike lesions, retinal arteritis, pale optic nerve head swelling, and localized segments of peripheral necrotizing retinitis. Visual acuity is not affected at this early stage, and sometimes this posterior involvement goes undetected if a dilated fundus examination of the peripheral retina is not performed. Unfortunately, if treatment is delayed for any reason, we may miss the only opportunity for successful therapy with acyclovir in an already affected eye.

In mild cases, the retinitis may not progress and may remain limited to less than 180 degrees of the peripheral retina. Approximately two-thirds of cases progress, however, and during the next 5 days the retinitis may extend to involve up to 360 degrees of the peripheral retina. Another characteristic of ARN is that it usually does not extend posterior to the vascular arcades, sparing the macula and thereby sparing central vision despite severe, extensive peripheral retinitis. In contrast to other forms of necrotizing retinitis such as cytomegalovirus retinitis or *Toxoplasma* retinitis, ARN progresses rapidly over a 7- to 10-day period and then stabilizes. The vitritis gradually increases and, in severe cases, the view of the retina may become compromised. During the most intense period of retinitis, an inferior exudative retinal detachment may occur temporarily.

Occasionally the peripheral visual field constricts, and there may be a sudden loss of central vision, even to no light perception, as a result of optic neuropathy. The causes of this optic neuropathy appear to be multifactorial, including inflammation, compression, and vasculitis. Even if vision falls to no light perception, some recovery may occur with high-dose steroids.

At any stage of the disease, central retinal vascular occlusion may occur, more often involving the central retinal artery than vein. Some cases even present with a central retinal artery or vein occlusion. Presumably, this results from the retinal vasculitis that affects both arteries and veins. Ando and colleagues [3], in 1982, discovered hyperaggregation of platelets, which probably contributes to retinal vascular occlusion.

Fluorescein angiography demonstrates both retinal and choroidal perfusion defects. Delayed and reduced retinal venous perfusion are seen, with sharp cut-off of fluorescein dye in areas of active retinitis.

The retinitis begins to resolve after approximately 3 weeks, or earlier with acyclovir treatment. The yellow-white retinitis recedes from its edges and from around retinal vessels, leaving atrophic retina in its wake. Vitritis increases during this phase as the necrotic retina sloughs into the vitreous cavity. Hard exudates representing residue of necrotic retina are sometimes found in areas of previous retinitis. The vitritis may decrease and visual acuity increase after resolution, deceiving some ophthalmologists and patients into thinking they are going to do well.

Unfortunately, rhegmatogenous retinal detachment may occur on an average of 65 days after the onset of the retinitis [4]. Retinal detachment is a result of the combined effects of large areas of full-thickness peripheral retinal necrosis and vitreous organization including preretinal and transvitreal traction. These detachments are complicated because of the vitreous organization and inflammation and the large posterior and multifocal retinal breaks.

ARN may affect the fellow eye in 20 to 70% of cases, usually within a month of the first eye. However, longer intervals are common, with up to 14 years being reported between eyes. There is no correlation between the severity of the disease in the first eye and that in the second eye.

Visual loss in ARN results primarily from retinal detachment, which occurs in 25 to 75% of cases. Optic neuropathy affects the vision in 10% and retinal vasculitis in 5%. Only rarely does the retinitis directly involve the macular area. Although early reports suggested that two-thirds of affected eyes had final visual acuities of 20/200 or worse [5], more recent studies indicate that only one-third of eyes have vision reduced to this level [6–8].

Matsuo and co-workers [9], in 1988, proposed that some cases of ARN were predestined to be mild, with limited peripheral retinitis, infrequent retinal detachment, and a good visual prognosis with or without treatment. Clearly there is a spectrum of disease severity from mild to severe cases, and any study that seeks to determine the efficacy of treatment modality must take into account this natural variation.

In the majority of cases of ARN, patients are otherwise systemically healthy and immunocompetent. A recent study by Usui [10], however, has shown a temporary decrease in delayed hypersensitivity by skin testing, although it is uncertain whether this represents cause or effect. Several reports have documented that ARN may occur after dermatomal herpes zoster dermatitis [11, 12]. This may involve the trigeminal nerve on the ipsilateral or contralateral side or may follow abdominal or thoracic herpes zoster infection [11]. A mild form of ARN may also follow systemic VZV infection or chickenpox. In addition, we have seen several cases in which adults develop ARN after close contact with a relative with chickenpox, although they did not exhibit any form of vesicular dermatitis. Many patients will give a history of recurrent fever blisters of the lips, presumably due to HSV. It should be emphasized, though, that most patients with ARN are healthy adults with no extraocular manifestations of a herpesvirus infection.

Although the majority of people with ARN are immunocompetent adults, typical cases of ARN have been seen in patients with AIDS or other types of immunocompromise. These patients usually are not completely immunoincompetent, generally having CD4 counts greater than 60. Most have a history of episodes of dermatomal herpes zoster or HSV dermatitis. The retinitis is typical in that it is rapidly progressive, peripheral, and responsive to acyclovir treatment. In patients with AIDS who have typical ARN, the disease tends to be severe and bilateral, with a poor visual outcome.

Laboratory Findings

Histopathological examination of 3 blind eyes that we enucleated during the active phase of ARN has demonstrated profound retinal necrosis sharply separated from normal retina by a junction zone of degenerating retinal cells containing intranuclear eosinophilic inclusions typical of herpesviruses. The retina and choroid are infiltrated by plasma cells and lymphocytes. The choroid is thickened by the infiltrate up to three times its normal thickness, underlying the areas of retinitis. The choriocapillaris is occluded only in the areas of retinitis. Localized areas of retinitis such as the posterior thumbprint lesions may histologically resemble a skin vesicle—that is, a retinal vesicle—with fused and lysed retinal cells in the vesicle (Fig 1).

There is diffuse retinal vasculitis particularly involving arterioles, which in some cases results in complete occlusion of the vascular lumen. Much of the retinal destruction in ARN appears to be the result of both retinal arteriolar and choriocapillaris occlusion. The optic nerve may be heavily infiltrated with inflammatory cells or may be infarcted. There is no evidence for direct viral infection of the optic nerve itself.

The viral origin of ARN was suspected in the early reports of Urayama, Kometani, Willerson, Young and their coauthors, but viral serological workup and pathological examination of inactive blind eyes failed to demonstrate a cause. ARN was originally believed to be an immunologically mediated vasculitis or uveitis. Consequently, many patients were treated with immunosuppressive agents with poor results. In 1982, we enucleated for diagnostic study a blind eye in a patient with bilateral ARN. Electron microscopy showed large quantities of a herpes type virus in the retina at the junction zone between necrotic and normal retina [13]. No virus was found in the choroid or the optic nerve. In 1985, we studied a blind eye that we had enucleated during the active phase of ARN from a healthy patient who had ARN in his other eye as well [14]. Again we found histopathological findings similar to the eye we had studied 3 years earlier, with necrotizing retinitis adjacent to unaffected retina. Viral cultures of the vitreous grew VZV, which was positively identified by DNA restriction enzyme analysis. We also studied the tissue from this eye and the previous

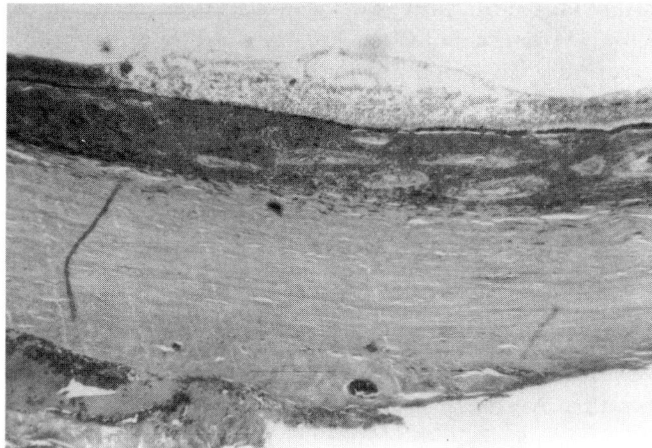

Figure 1 *Retinal vesicle corresponding to posterior thumbprintlike lesions, with fused and lysed retinal cells in the vesicle similar to skin vesicles in herpes simplex or varicella zoster dermatitis.*

eye immunocytologically using the avidin-biotin-peroxidase technique. VZV antigens were found in both specimens in the transition zone between normal and necrotic retina in both neuroretinal and retinal pigment epithelium. Antigen was not detected in the choroid, ciliary body, vascular endothelium, or optic nerve. This correlated with the electron-microscopical findings. Thus, we confirmed in 2 different cases that VZV was a cause of ARN.

HSV continued to be suspected as a cause of ARN as well. In 1987, we treated a patient with bilateral ARN who was not responding well to acyclovir treatment [15]. We performed a diagnostic vitrectomy in the worst eye and recovered HSV type I on viral culture. Thus, it was confirmed that HSV type I as well as VZV could cause ARN. Since then, Ganley and Zimmerman have described cases of ARN that were suspected to be caused by HSV type II, but isolation of HSV II directly from the eye in a case of ARN has not yet been accomplished.

■ Primary Versus Reactivated Viral ARN

In the cases of VZV and HSV ARN just cited, clinical and serological data indicated that the patients had acquired their respective viral infections earlier in life either as chickenpox or herpes simplex vesicular dermatitis. Thus, these cases represent reactivated latent herpesvirus.

It appears that retinitis may follow primary infections as well [15–17]. A mild type of ARN follows primary chickenpox rarely, with limited retinitis, unilateral involvement, and good visual results. We have isolated HSV type I from the vitreous of a healthy 20-year-old patient who had a diffuse fulminating retinitis involving the entire retina that appeared to be occurring during the course of a primary HSV-I infection [15].

Thus, HSV and VZV cause ARN both as recurrent secondary infections or, rarely, as primary infections. Typical ARN appears to occur in healthy patients as a secondary reactivation of previously acquired latent virus. Atypical mild ARN occurs occasionally following chickenpox—that is, a primary VZV infection. Severe diffuse, fulminant retinitis is seen during the course of primary HSV infections.

Factors Influencing Patient Susceptibility and Disease Severity

Hara [18] and Matsuo [19] and their colleagues have reviewed the clinical features of cases of ARN to determine whether any early characteristics could be used to predict the final visual outcome. They found that the more extensive and rapidly progressive the retinitis, the worse the visual prognosis. Other poor prognostic factors found by Matsuo were a reduced electroretinogram, extensive retinal arteritis, and high levels of circulating immune complexes.

Usui [10] recently reported a study of 32 ARN eyes in which he determined the causative virus by comparing the level of antibody for HSV and VZV in the aqueous and in the serum. His investigations revealed some interesting differences in the clinical patterns of ARN caused by HSV and VZV. ARN caused by VZV occurred in older persons with mutton-fat keratic precipitates and was more extensive, with retinal arteritis, a higher frequency of retinal detachment, and a poorer visual prognosis. ARN caused by HSV occurred in younger patients and was less extensive, with less frequent retinal detachments, a better visual prognosis, and less likelihood for bilaterality. Usui [10] also found that VZV ARN tended to occur in the spring of the year, whereas HSV ARN occurred more often in the winter. These findings are similar to the differences in age of onset and the seasons of onset for herpes zoster ophthalmicus and herpes simplex keratitis.

Clearly, ARN is a disease with a spectrum of severity, varying from mild cases with limited retinitis and good visual results to severe cases with extensive retinitis and a poor visual result. In Matsuo's recent study [19], affected eyes had either a good final best-corrected visual acuity or an extremely poor final visual acuity, with very few cases at intermediate levels of visual reduction. This is because the disease typically spares the macula and, if the retina does not detach and if there is no central vascular occlusion or significant optic neuropathy, the visual result will be good.

In addition to the species of the virus, other factors presumably play a role in determining the severity of the disease. These include the neurovirulent properties of the individual virus, which can vary tremendously from one HSV to another. Probably the most important difference is whether ARN is caused by HSV or VZV.

Another factor that may affect patient susceptibility to the disease as well as the severity of the disease is the host immunogenetic response pattern. In the United States, in Caucasian patients, Holland and associates [20] have detected a significantly higher frequency of HLA-DQw7 and phenotype Bw62, DR4 in ARN patients than in the general population. Ichikaw and associates [21] found an association of ARN with Aw33, B-44, and DRw6 either alone or in combination in Japanese patients. The fact that ARN syndrome may be associated with HLA-DR4 in Caucasian patients and HLA-DR6 in Japanese patients suggests that the disease predisposition is associated with the same region of DNA; HLA-DR4 and HLA-DR6 are encoded in the same region that controls positions 69 through 72 of the first domain of the HLA-DR molecule. In addition to this HLA-determined predisposition to ARN, Matsuo and co-workers [19] have shown that the severe type of ARN tends to be associated with HLA-DRw9. Thus, both susceptibility to ARN and disease severity may, in part, be determined by the patient's immunogenetic structure.

Treatment

Progress in the treatment of ARN has been slow despite considerable knowledge regarding its clinical course, herpesvirus etiology, and theoretically effective antiviral therapy. For purposes of discussion, the treatment of ARN may be separated into that which has become generally accepted and that which should still be considered controversial.

Based on the knowledge that ARN is caused by either VZV or HSV, acyclovir is the current choice for antiviral treatment of active ARN. In ARN, acyclovir is given as early as possible, intravenously, at a dose of 500 mg/m^2 every 8 hours for 10 days. Usually the retinitis begins to regress after 5 days of treatment [4], although several weeks may elapse before the retinitis has resolved completely. After a 10-day course of intravenous administration, oral acyclovir is given at a dose of 800 mg five times daily for 3 months.

The beneficial effects of acyclovir in ARN that have been proved include a fivefold decrease in the risk of involvement of the fellow eye, from approximately 70 to 13%, as determined by a multicenter retrospective study by Palay and colleagues [22]. In addition, acyclovir treatment appears to curtail the retinitis, with early regression beginning, on average, within 5 days of treatment [4].

There is no study to date which demonstrates that the rate of retinal detachment or the final visual acuity is affected by acyclovir treatment. Viral isolates of both HSV and VZV have been sensitive in vitro to acyclovir at the levels that we expect to be present in the vitreous in ARN. However, all these isolates were recovered from eyes while patients were receiving intravenous acyclovir treatment. Because treatment of ARN usually is begun long after the retinitis is well established, it may be that all the retinal cells that are going to be infected by virus have already been infected early in the course of the disease but have not yet become opaque or necrotic. Thus, even with acyclovir treatment, the retinitis may appear to progress for a period, although acyclovir may actually be preventing new infection of uninfected cells. Support for this theory comes from the mouse model for HSV retinitis in which virus may be detected in retinal cells several days before the retina becomes opaque or necrotic. Possibly, we could influence the disease more with acyclovir if we could begin treatment on the very first day that retinitis appears. Unfortunately, by the time the diagnosis of ARN is made, the retinitis has presumably been present for days or even weeks. Nonetheless, acyclovir treatment should be given, if only to decrease the risk of bilateral involvement.

Corticosteroids are administered along with acyclovir to decrease the severe intraocular inflammation encountered in ARN. These may be given as high-dose oral or intravenous drugs. Periocular depot steroids and topical steroid drops may also be used, especially to suppress vitreous and anterior segment inflammation. In a case of severe ARN, either 100 mg prednisone orally every day or 250 mg methylprednisolone intravenously four times daily may be given, particularly if there is evidence of severe optic neuropathy. For mild cases, lower-dose oral steroids such as 40 mg prednisone and topical steroid drops may be adequate antiinflammatory treatment.

As stated earlier, Ando and associates [3] have reported the hyperaggregation of platelets in ARN, and vascular obstruction has been demonstrated by fluorescein angiography and histopathological examination. Therefore, antiplatelet therapy with aspirin, 30 mg/day, has been advocated in the hope of decreasing the vasoocclusive component of this disease, although the efficacy of this treatment is uncertain.

Prophylactic laser photocoagulation is now used routinely in an attempt to prevent the complication of rhegmatogenous retinal detachment. Confluent rows of photocoagulation are applied posterior to the areas of active retinitis, theoretically to create a "new" ora serrata. Studies by Sternberg [6] and Han [7] and their colleagues appear to document the value of prophylactic photocoagulation when compared to an untreated control group. However, in both studies, the control and treatment groups were not comparable because the treated group consisted primarily of mild cases with limited retinitis, which were treatable because they had minimal vitritis. Our experience is that photocoagulation does not prevent retinal detachment in severe ARN, which is the most likely setting for detachment. The mild cases are less likely to detach, although photocoagulation may prevent retinal detachment in some of those mild cases in which detachment may have occurred. There appears to be no harm in applying prophylactic photocoagulation and thus it is probably indicated. It should be employed as soon as the retinitis stabilizes before the vitreous becomes too cloudy to permit photocoagulation of the retina.

Prophylactic surgery to prevent retinal detachment has been considered and even advocated by some clinicians because of the high incidence of retinal detachment particularly in severe cases. Surgical intervention involves pars plana vitrectomy, photocoagulation, scleral buckles, and intraocular antiviral agents. The timing of operation is difficult to determine because of the presence of severe intraocular inflammation during the active phase of ARN, before rhegmatogenous retinal detachment develops. The only other situation in which pars plana vitrectomy is performed on as severely inflamed eyes as these is in endophthalmitis. Clearly, this surgery is *not* indicated in mild cases of ARN.

Rhegmatogenous retinal detachments that occur after ARN are difficult to repair because of (1) the multiplicity and posterior location of retinal breaks, which make selection of an appropriate scleral buckle difficult; (2) the presence of vitreous traction and proliferative vitreoretinopathy; and (3) the inflammatory nature of the disease, which results in a high rate of postoperative complications, such as an acute fibrinous response and choroidal detachment.

The 1984 study by Clarkson and associates [23] from the Bascom Palmer Eye Institute reported a 50% incidence of retinal detachment, two-thirds of which were successfully reattached. A later report in 1989 by the same group, using currently available vitreoretinal techniques of vitrectomy-lensectomy, endolaser, internal drainage, and tamponade demonstrated an improved anatomical reattachment rate of 94% [8]. Scleral buckling is controversial given the potential for anterior segment ischemia, choroidal detachment, glaucoma or hypotony, and increased intraocular fibrin formation.

■ Rapidly Progressive Outer Retinal Necrosis

There are two other acute retinitis syndromes caused by HSV and VZV that are distinct from ARN but that share some common features. The first, termed *rapidly progressive outer retinal necrosis* [24, 25], occurs in the latest stages of AIDS and is characterized by bilateral, rapidly progressive, deep retinitis with minimal evidence of vitritis or retinal vasculitis (Fig 2). It presents with multifocal deep retinal lesions that progress to involve the superficial retina, eventually becoming confluent and spreading throughout the entire retina.

VZV has been isolated from eyes affected with this syndrome. In contrast to ARN, the posterior pole may be involved, sometimes with a cherry-red macula. The disorder appears to be relatively resistant to acyclovir treatment, and almost all eyes eventually become blind.

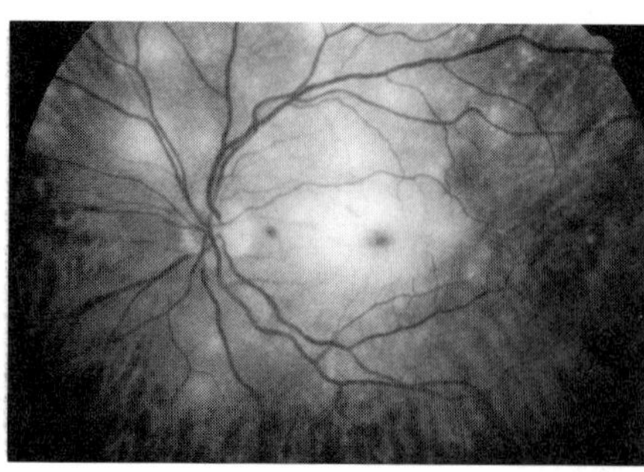

Figure 2 *Rapidly progressive outer retinal necrosis caused by varicella zoster virus in the late stages of the acquired immunodeficiency syndrome. Minimal vitritis is present. Many eyes have early macular involvement followed by peripheral and then diffuse retinitis.*

■ Diffuse Fulminant Herpetic Retinitis

Diffuse fulminant herpetic retinitis is characterized by a fulminant necrotizing retinitis that diffusely destroys the entire retina, including the macula, in a few days. HSV causes this disorder in one of two settings: either acute retinitis occurring in a nonimmune person as a primary, first-time infection [15] or during the course of HSV encephalitis presumably by spread down the optic nerve to the eye. Both of these clinical presentations are very uncommon.

■ Comparison of Three Acute Retinitis Syndromes

A comparison of these three syndromes—ARN, rapidly progressive outer retinal necrosis, and diffuse fulminant herpetic retinitis—provides insight into how their differing immune and inflammatory responses produce their differing clinical pictures. In ARN, the virus may spread to the peripheral retina, where it stimulates a marked inflammatory response but is contained there because of intact effective immune resistance to the virus. In rapidly progressive outer retinal necrosis, although the patient had previous immunity to the virus, his or her AIDS is so advanced that he or she cannot respond immunologically and cannot mount an inflammatory response. Thus, the VZV infection progresses relentlessly with no intraocular inflammation. In diffuse fulminant herpetic retinitis, the patient has no prior immunity to the virus but is able to mount a normal inflammatory response to foreign viral invasion. Thus, the herpetic retinitis progresses without immune interference but with marked inflammation as it rapidly destroys the entire retina.

■ Animal Models of ARN

Acute necrotizing retinitis, which shares many features with ARN in humans, can be induced experimentally in rabbits and mice. In 1924, von

Szily [26] reported that injection of HSV into one eye of a rabbit produces retinal necrosis in the uninoculated, contralateral eye [26], a finding that recently was duplicated in mice [27].

After uniocular anterior chamber inoculation of HSV type I, between 70 and 100% of the mice developed progressive necrotizing retinitis in the contralateral eye, characterized by inflammation in all layers of the retina, vasculitis, hemorrhage, schisis and, finally, loss of the retinal architecture [27]. Acute retinitis proceeds rapidly to retinal necrosis, often within 24 hours. In mice, the anterior segment of the uninoculated eye exhibits mild iridocyclitis, but viral infection of the anterior segment does not occur. In the injected eye, the pattern of involvement is reversed. In this eye, there is massive inflammation of the anterior segment and, although retinal folding and mild to moderate vitritis are observed in the posterior segment, the retina of the inoculated eye is not infected with virus and is not necrotic [27–29]. Some aspects of the mouse model of HSV type I ARN parallel those observed in human patients with ARN, namely: (1) rapid retinal destruction by a herpesvirus; (2) occurrence in immunocompetent, healthy mice; and (3) subclinical involvement of the central nervous system (CNS). These similarities between the mouse model of ARN and what has been observed in human patients with ARN have led to further investigations using the mouse model that may eventually increase our understanding of the pathogenesis of ARN in human patients.

The optic nerve has been shown to be the conduit by which the virus is transmitted to the retina of the uninoculated eye [30]. Recent studies have defined the route of spread of the virus from the injected eye through the CNS to the uninoculated eye. Although it was initially hypothesized that virus entered the CNS via the optic nerve of the injected eye, our recent experiments and those of other investigators have demonstrated, after anterior chamber inoculation of HSV type I, that virus leaves the injected eye by two non–optic nerve routes: the trigeminal sensory nerves that supply the anterior segment and the parasympathetic fibers of the oculomotor nerve that supply the iris and the ciliary body [31, 32] (Fig 3).

The first route to the CNS via the trigeminal nerves allows virus to reach the trigeminal ganglion. Once in the ganglion, however, virus is unable to spread into the second-order sensory neurons of the nucleus of the spinal trigeminal tract in the brain stem. The second route by which virus leaves the injected eye is the parasympathetic component of the third cranial nerve, and virus is first detected in the ipsilateral ciliary ganglion at 48 hours postinjection (p.i.). From the ciliary ganglion, virus travels via axonal transport to the ipsilateral Edinger-Westphal nucleus and from there to the suprachiasmatic nuclei of the hypothalamus and the visual system. We hypothesize that the timing of virus spread from the Edinger-Westphal nucleus to the suprachiasmatic nuclei is critically important in determining whether one or both retinas will be affected. Virus is detected in the ipsilateral suprachiasmatic nucleus of virus-infected mice at day 5 postinjection, but the virus is not detected in the contralateral suprachias-

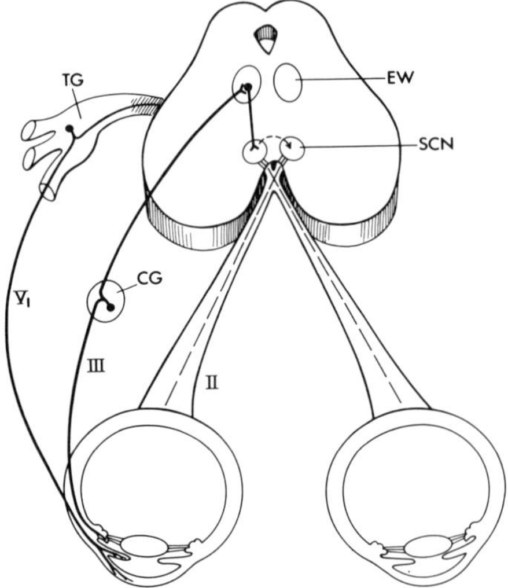

Figure 3 *The two pathways of viral spread after inoculation of virus into the anterior chamber of a mouse. Spread of virus via the first pathway, the ophthalmic division of the trigeminal nerve* (V_1), *results in either initial establishment of latency or return to latency in the trigeminal ganglion (TG). Spread of virus by the oculomotor nerve (III) pathway through the ciliary ganglion (CG) to the Edinger-Westphal (EW) nucleus is followed by spread of virus to the ipsilateral suprachiasmatic nucleus (SCN) and the contralateral optic nerve (II). Spread of virus from the ipsilateral SCN to the contralateral SCN would allow virus to reach both optic nerves and both retinas.*

matic nucleus until day 7 postinjection. On or near this same day, virus reaches the optic nerve of the contralateral eye by direct spread from the ipsilateral suprachiasmatic nucleus. In contrast, virus apparently is unable to enter the ipsilateral optic nerve from the contralateral suprachiasmatic nucleus [32]. The difference in timing of virus entry into the suprachiasmatic nuclei may explain why infected mice develop necrotizing retinitis only in the uninoculated eye: One reason mice infected with virus do not have retinal necrosis in the inoculated eye may be because the host's immune response to the virus is established in time for virus-specific immune effector modalities to limit viral spread from the contralateral suprachiasmatic nucleus into the optic nerve of the injected eye.

These results also suggest that specific immune effector mechanisms or antiviral therapies are likely to be limited in what they can accomplish in individuals with ARN. In mice and in human patients with ARN after primary infection by the virus, the host's own immune response may be mobilized too late for it to have any effect on the spread of the virus. In patients with ARN due to viral reactivation, preexisting antiviral immunity may be insufficient to prevent viral replication and spread from the site of latency. In addition, there may be a problem related to accessibility of immune effector modalities as virus spreads from the site of reactivation to an ocular site; virus transported to the eye via axonal transport may not be accessible to either cellular or humoral immune effector mechanisms in the early stages of the reactivated disease. Furthermore, these results suggest that for any antiviral therapy to be effective in ARN, such therapy should be administered early in the course of the disease before the onset of retinal symptoms. However, as previously discussed, this is difficult because, by the time the retinal symptoms occur in patients with ARN, the viral infection is well established.

Knowledge of routes of viral spread from the mouse model may provide insight into the mechanism of ARN in humans. Many patients with ARN have anterior uveitis, and most also have evidence of optic nerve involvement. By extrapolation from the mouse, we hypothesize that the following sequence of events might occur in human ARN:

1. Herpesvirus infection results in mild anterior uveitis, as a result of either a primary or a reactivated infection from the corresponding trigeminal ganglion. The site of primary or reactivated infection may be either on the cornea (which can result in infection of anterior segment structures) or within the eye.
2. Once on the cornea or in the anterior segment, probably in the vast majority of eyes with herpetic anterior uveitis the disease resolves, and the virus returns to latency in the trigeminal ganglion.
3. In patients destined to develop ARN, the virus does not become latent in the trigeminal ganglion but instead travels via the parasympathetic component of the oculomotor nerve to the CNS.
4. Once the virus reaches the CNS, it enters the optic pathway of one or both eyes following the route described for the mouse model and then travels to the retina via the optic nerve.

As in the mouse, it is possible that in humans the virus may be arrested at one of several sites in the CNS either by cell-mediated immune mechanisms or by antibody of sufficiently high titer and affinity. The development of ARN in human patients might therefore be viewed as a failure of the host to control either a primary or a reactivated infection with herpesvirus.

■ Future Directions

Other aspects about human ARN that remain to be elucidated include the following:

1. Why occasionally is there such a long lag between the development of ARN in one eye and the other?
2. Why is the peripheral retina mainly involved? (We would suggest that perhaps there are fibers in the suprachiasmatic nucleus that are more susceptible to viral infection, and perhaps those fibers supply the peripheral retina in humans.)
3. Can HSV or VZV become latent in CNS structures other than the trigeminal ganglion?

In the 20 years since Urayama's original description [1], we have learned a great deal about ARN, including its herpesvirus causation, the spectrum of clinical severity, the beneficial effects of acyclovir treatment, and the techniques for repair of its associated retinal detachments. The pathogenesis of the disease, however, remains uncertain, and existing medical treatment still does not prevent the severe sequelae in an already affected eye.

■ References

1. Urayama A, Yamada N, Sasaki T, et al. Unilateral acute uveitis with retinal periarteritis and detachment. Jpn J Clin Ophthalmol 1971;25:607–619
2. Young NJ, Bird AC. Bilateral acute retinal necrosis. Br J Ophthalmol 1978;62:581–590
3. Ando F, Goto S, Kato M, et al. Platelet function in six cases of Kirisawa's uveitis. Folia Ophthalmol Jpn 1982;33:976–982
4. Blumenkranz MS, Culbertson WW, Clarkson JG, Dix R. Treatment of the acute retinal necrosis syndrome with intravenous acyclovir. Ophthalmology 1986;93:296–300
5. Fisher JP, Lewis ML, Blumenkranz MS, et al. The acute retinal necrosis syndrome. Part I. clinical manifestations. Ophthalmology 1982;89:1309–1316
6. Sternberg P Jr, Han DP, Yeo JH, et al. Photocoagulation to prevent retinal detachment in acute retinal necrosis. Ophthalmology 1988;95:1389–1393
7. Han DP, Lewis H, Williams GA, et al. Laser photocoagulation in the acute retinal necrosis syndrome. Arch Ophthalmol 1987;105:1051–1054
8. Blumenkranz M, Clarkson J, Culbertson WW, et al. Vitrectomy for retinal detachment associated with acute retinal necrosis. Am J Ophthalmol 1988;106:426–429
9. Matsuo T, Nakayama T, Koyama T, et al. A proposed mild type of acute retinal necrosis syndrome. Am J Ophthalmol 1988;105:579–583
10. Usui M. Clinical differences in the pattern of Kirisawa-Urayama uveitis induced by different herpes viruses. Jpn Rev Clin Ophthalmol 1991;85:868–875
11. Browning DJ, Blumenkranz MS, Culbertson WW, et al. Association of varicella zoster dermatitis with acute retinal necrosis syndrome. Ophthalmology 1987;94:602–606
12. Yeo JH, Pepose JS, Stewart JA, et al. Acute retinal necrosis syndrome following herpes zoster dermatitis. Ophthalmology 1986;93:1418–1422
13. Culbertson WW, Blumenkranz MS, Haines H, et al. The acute retinal necrosis syndrome. II. Histopathology and etiology. Ophthalmology 1982;89:1317–1325
14. Culbertson WW, Blumenkranz MS, Pepose JS, et al. Varicella zoster is a cause of the acute retinal necrosis syndrome. Ophthalmology 1986;93:559–568
15. Lewis ML, Culbertson WW, Post JD, et al. Herpes simplex virus type I; a cause of the acute retinal necrosis syndrome. Ophthalmology 1989;96:875–878
16. Matsuo T, Koyama M, Umezv H, Matsuo N. Acute retinal necrosis developing after chickenpox in adults. Jpn J Clin Ophthalmol 1990;44:605–607
17. Culbertson WW, Brod RD, Flynn HW Jr, et al. Chickenpox associated acute retinal necrosis syndrome. Ophthalmology 1991;98:1642–1646
18. Hara Y, Nakagawa Y, Tada R, et al. Clinical features of 31 cases of Kirisawa-type uveitis. Jpn J Clin Ophthalmol 1990;44:663–666
19. Matsuo T, Morimoto K, Matsuo N. Factors associated with poor visual outcome in acute retinal necrosis. Br J Ophthalmol 1991;75:450–454

20. Holland GN, Cornell PJ, Park MS, et al. An association between acute retinal necrosis syndrome and HLA-DQw7 and phenotype Bw 62, DR4. Am J Ophthalmol 1989;108:370–374
21. Ichikaw T, Sakai J, Usui M, et al. HLA antigens of patients with Kirisawa's uveitis and herpetic keratitis. J Eye 1989;6:107–114
22. Palay DA, Sternberg P Jr, Davis J, et al. Decrease in the risk of bilateral acute retinal necrosis by acyclovir therapy. Am J Ophthalmol 1991;112:250–255
23. Clarkson JG, Blumenkranz MS, Culbertson WW, et al. Retinal detachment following the acute retinal necrosis syndrome. Ophthalmology 1984;91:1665–1668
24. Forster DJ, Dugel PU, Frangieh GT, et al. Rapidly progressive outer retinal necrosis in the acquired immunodeficiency syndrome. Am J Ophthalmol 1990;110:341–348
25. Margolis TP, Lowder CY, Holland GN. Varicella-zoster retinitis in patients with the acquired immunodeficiency syndrome. Am J Ophthalmol 1991;112:119–131
26. von Szily A. An experimental endogenous transmission of infection from bulbus to bulbus. Klin Monatsbl Augenheilkd 1924;75:593–602
27. Whittum JA, McCulley JP, Niederkorn JY, Streilein JW. Ocular disease induced in mice by anterior chamber inoculation of herpes simplex virus. Invest Ophthalmol Vis Sci 1984;25:1065–1073
28. Cousins SW, Altman NH, Atherton SS. Schisis contributes to necrosis in experimental HSV-1 retinitis. Exp Eye Res 1989;48:745–760
29. Cousins SW, Gonzalez AR, Atherton SS. Herpes simplex retinitis in the mouse: clinicopathologic correlations. Invest Ophthalmol Vis Sci 1989;30:1485–1494
30. Bosem ME, Harris R, Atherton SS. Optic nerve involvement in viral spread in herpes simplex virus type 1 retinitis. Invest Ophthalmol Vis Sci 1990;31:1683–1689
31. Margolis TP, LaVail J, Setzer PY, Dawson CR. Selective spread of herpes simplex virus in the central nervous system after ocular inoculation. J Virol 1989;63:4756–4761
32. Vann VR, Atherton SS. Neural spread of herpes simplex virus after anterior chamber inoculation. Invest Ophthalmol Vis Sci 1991;32:2462–2472

Ocular Microsporidiosis

Careen Yen Lowder, M.D., Ph.D.

Microsporidia are intracellular spore-forming protozoan parasites found worldwide and known to infect most major animal groups, vertebrate and invertebrate. Prior to reports of human infections, extensive studies of microsporidia resulted from the economic impact of parasitism by microsporidia in insects such as the silkworm, honeybees, and other animal groups such as fish [1]. The first well-documented case of microsporidian infection in humans was reported in 1959: A Japanese boy exposed to farm animals presented with headache, convulsions, and recurrent fever. Examination of the cerebrospinal fluid revealed organisms identified as microsporidia, genus *Encephalitozoon* [2]. The next two reports were in 1973: An immunocompromised infant with thymic aplasia died of severe diarrhea and malabsorption. The microsporidia *Nosema connori* were identified in most organs including lungs, diaphragm, stomach, intestines, kidneys, liver, and heart [3]. The other report was of corneal involvement in an 11-year-old boy from Sri Lanka [4]. A second report of corneal infection appeared in 1981 and involved a 26-year-old woman from Botswana [5]. In 1984, a 3-year-old Colombian boy adopted by a Swedish family developed seizures and hepatomegaly. The microsporidian *Encephalitozoon cuniculi* was identified as the causative organism [6]. In 1985, a 20-year-old black man with progressive generalized muscle weakness was found, after two sets of muscle biopsies, to be infected with microsporidia of the genus *Pleistophora* [7].

Between 1959 and 1990, only 8 cases of human microsporidiosis had been reported in the immunocompetent or immunocompromised individual without the acquired immunodeficiency syndrome (AIDS). Four of these cases involved the eye [4, 5, 8, 9]. Since 1985, more than 60 cases of microsporidian infections have been reported in patients with chronic diarrhea, malabsorption, and AIDS [10]. The first case of AIDS-related microsporidian hepatitis appeared in 1987, and a case of peritonitis was reported in 1989 [11, 12]. Since 1990, 7 cases of microsporidian corneal infections in AIDS patients have been reported [9, 13–16].

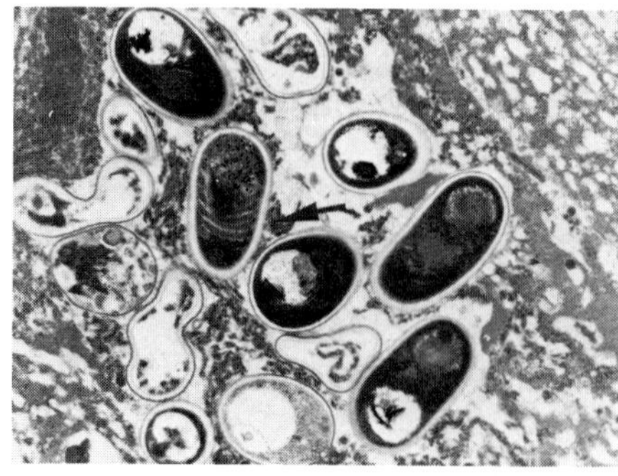

Figure 1 *Transmission electron micrograph of microsporidian spores. The organisms are characterized by a coiled polar tubule (arrow) (×24,000). (Reprinted with permission from Lowder et al [13]. Copyright by the Ophthalmic Publishing Company.)*

■ Causative Organisms in Microsporidiosis

The order Microsporidia is found within the phylum Microspora. The coiled polar tubule is the principal feature used to distinguish microsporidia from other protozoa (Fig 1). Four genera have been implicated in human disease: *Encephalitozoon, Nosema, Enterocytozoon,* and *Pleistophora.* Several features distinguish and place microsporidian organisms in the appropriate genus: Among the genera and species there is variation in the number of coils, the size of the spore, the number and configuration of nuclei in the spores, and the relationship between the parasite and host cell (the presence or absence of a parasitophorous vacuole formed either by the host cell or the parasite) [1].

Enterocytozoon

The genus *Enterocytozoon* has been implicated in all documented cases of intestinal microsporidiosis in patients with AIDS [9]. The organism is characterized by a polar tubule and develops in direct contact with host cell cytoplasm (not within a vacuole).

Pleistophora

Pleistophora is found in the skeletal muscles of fish. In 1985, Ledford and colleagues [7] reported *Pleistophora* in the skeletal muscles of a 20-year-old black man with muscle weakness. *Pleistophora* is characterized by a parasite-formed parasitophorous vacuole.

Nosema

The genus *Nosema* is characterized by oval parasite spores measuring 4 × 2 μm. Electron microscopy reveals 10 or more coils of the polar tubule, 2 nuclei in diplokaryon arrangement (paired nuclei), and spores in direct contact with the host cell cytoplasm (absence of a vacuole) [1].

Encephalitozoon

The first infection by *Encephalitozoon* was reported in a 9-year-old Japanese boy [2]. The patient was treated for 3 months with sulfisoxazole for fever, loss of consciousness, headache, and convulsions, and was then discharged in good condition. The genus *Encephalitozoon* is characterized by small spore size (approximately 1 × 2 μm), five to seven coils of the polar tubule, proliferative cells that contain an isolated nucleus (no diplokaryon), and the presence of a host-produced parasitophorous vacuole [1].

■ Ocular Microsporidiosis

Clinical Findings

There are two distinct clinical presentations of ocular microsporidiosis, each of which depends on the immune status of the host. A corneal stromal keratitis is seen in immunocompetent patients, whereas an epithelial keratopathy is seen in patients with AIDS.

Corneal Stromal Keratitis Four cases of microsporidian keratitis have been reported in immunocompetent individuals. The first reports of ocular infections by microsporidia were attributed to *Nosema.* In 1973, a boy from Sri Lanka was gored by a goat in the right eye, leading to corneal scarring [4]. Six years later, he developed keratitis. A biopsy of the cornea revealed a necrotic central stroma surrounded by acute inflammatory cells. Immediately above Descemet's membrane were many oval bodies. Because the nucleation was not observed, the genus designation was not proved. Canning and Lom [17] recently transferred this parasite into the genus *Microsporidium ceylonensis.*

The second case of microsporidian keratitis was described in a 26-year-old woman from Botswana, Africa, in 1981, who presented with a perforated corneal ulcer in her left eye without prior history of trauma [5]. The keratitis was unresponsive to treatment, and the eye was enucleated. Histopathological examination revealed the cornea to be infiltrated with neutrophils, mononuclear cells, epithelioid granulomas, and many oval organisms. Electron-microscopical analyses revealed spores containing a polar tubule that made 11 to 13 coils and parasites that were free in the host cell. Although the authors classified the organisms as *Nosema* species, because of the lack of information on the nuclear arrangements, this parasite was transferred into the genus *M. africanum* [17].

Since 1990, 2 additional cases of microsporidian corneal infection were reported in the immunocompetent patient. One patient, a 45-year-old man from South Carolina, presented with decreased vision in his left eye [8]. The initial examination revealed a small central area of epithelial irregularity and a midstromal infiltrate associated with stromal edema. An iritis was present. Over the next 11 months, the patient was treated with topical prednisolone acetate 1% and neomycin-bacitracin-polymyxin eye drops. The stromal infiltrate slowly enlarged, and central corneal biopsy was performed 11 months after presentation. The stromal infiltrate continued to enlarge and, when it reached approximately 8 mm in diameter 23 months after presentation, the patient had a penetrating keratoplasty. Histopathological examination revealed large numbers of spores, intact stromal lamellae, and lack of an inflammatory cellular reaction. Organisms recovered from the corneal biopsy and keratoplasty specimen have been successfully recovered in vitro [18]. The spores measured 3.7 × 1 μm, had two nuclei (diplokaryon), and replicated in the host cytoplasm; the polar tubule coiled five to six turns. Because of the different morphological characteristics from previously described *Nosema* species, the authors have named the organism *Nosema corneum*.

The other case involved a 39-year-old man from Ohio who developed blurred vision and irritation in his left eye. A foreign body was removed but the corneal ulcer persisted. A biopsy of the persistent corneal inflammatory bed revealed microsporidian organisms [9].

Corneal Epithelial Keratopathy   Reports of microsporidian keratitis in patients with AIDS first appeared in 1990. Six cases have since been reported in the United States and, recently, 1 case was reported in Great Britain [9, 13–16]. All 7 cases shared similar symptoms and clinical findings. In cases where biopsy specimens were obtained, there were similar histopathological features. Patients present with redness, foreign-body sensation, blurred vision, and photophobia. Slit-lamp examination reveals conjunctival hyperemia, minimal or no inflammatory response and, in advanced cases, lack of conjunctival luster. The cornea is seen to have a coarse punctate epithelial keratopathy (Fig 2). Conjunctival and corneal scrapings demonstrate a large number of microsporidian spores and few or no inflammatory cells. Electron microscopy demonstrates spores measuring 1 × 2 μm; the polar tubule forms six to eight coiled loops around

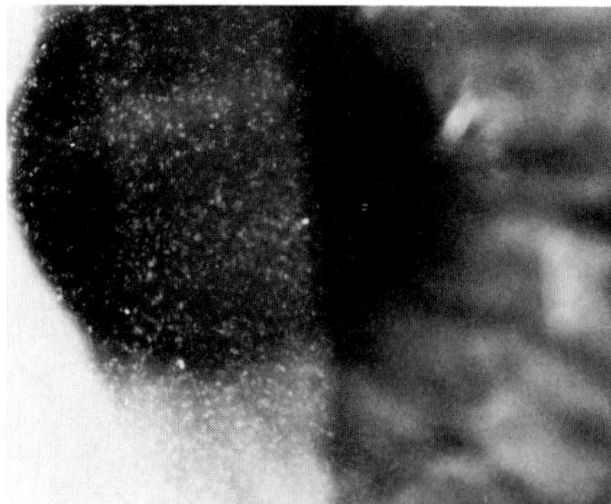

Figure 2   *Slit-lamp photograph reveals coarse punctate epithelial keratopathy. (Reprinted with permission from Lowder et al [13]. Copyright by the Ophthalmic Publishing Company.)*

a single nucleus. Three of the reported cases were from New York: All were infected with *Encephalitozoon hellen*. *E. hellen* and *E. cuniculi* have a similar morphological appearance but different polyacrylamide gel electrophoresis protein profiles [19]. Two cases involved *Encephalitozoon*-like organisms [19, 20]. In the case from Ohio [13], the patient's punctate epithelial keratopathy progressed despite treatment with many antimicrobial agents. The keratopathy became confluent with development of severe corneal vascularization, while the conjunctiva acquired a dry and irregular appearance.

Diagnosis

The microsporidian organism is difficult to recover in culture. Diagnosis of microsporidiosis requires identification of the distinctive coiled polar tubule by electron microscopy of biopsy specimens. The increasing numbers of reports of human microsporidiosis may be secondary to increased awareness of the disease. In the examination of corneal tissues, microsporidian spores are gram-positive. A single body that stains positively for periodic acid–Schiff may be seen at one end of the oval body, but routine hematoxylin and eosin staining fails to visualize the organisms. Staining of microsporidia with Gomori's methenamine silver (GMS) fungus stain, acid-fast stain, and Giemsa stain is variable. Reliable serological tests are not currently available for the diagnosis of microsporidiosis [19].

Treatment

No effective treatment is known for human microsporidiosis. Sulfisoxazole, alone or in combination with trimethoprim, and chloroquine have been used with variable results [2, 6, 7, 9]. Ocular microsporidiosis in the immunocompetent patient has led to loss of the eye and a failed corneal graft in early reports. In the case reported in 1990, the stromal disease was most likely modified and decreased by the use of topical corticosteroids [8]. This patient had a penetrating keratoplasty without recurrence of microsporidiosis.

In patients with AIDS, reports of successful treatment with a combination of antibiotics and antiparasitic agents have usually been followed by recurrence of infection. Yee and co-workers [15] reported resolution of microsporidian keratitis in a patient who was on itraconazole, a new triazole antifungal agent, for cryptococcal meningitis. Metcalfe and associates [16] reported resolution of microsporidian keratoconjunctivitis in a patient treated with propamidine isethionate 0.1%; however, the infection recurred when the drug was discontinued. Fumagillin and chloroquine are effective against *E. cuniculi* in vitro, and fumagillin is used in the treatment of infected honeybees [1].

Transmission

Transmission of microsporidia is usually through the oral-fecal route. Trauma and proximity to the tropics have been implicated in the development of microsporidiosis. In patients with ocular disease, direct inoculation is postulated. Of the 7 patients with AIDS, 4 were known to have domestic pets, and these pets may have been the infectious source.

■ Conclusion

Microsporidiosis is increasingly reported as an opportunistic infection in patients with AIDS. Although only 4 cases of ocular microsporidiosis were reported between 1973 and 1990 in immunocompetent individuals, 7 cases of microsporidian keratopathy have been reported since 1990 in patients with AIDS. The two distinct clinical presentations of ocular microsporidiosis implicate the host's immune response in the severity of disease observed in the immunocompetent host. With the increasing incidence of microsporidiosis in humans, studies should aim at finding treatment modalities.

■ References

1. Cali A, Owen R. Microsporidiosis. In: Balows A, Hausler WJ, eds. The laboratory diagnosis of infectious diseases: principles and practice, vol 1. New York: Springer-Verlag, 1988:929–950
2. Matsubayashi H, Koike T, Mikata T, Hagiwara S. A case of *Encephalitozoon*-like body infection in man. Arch Pathol 1959;67:181–187
3. Margileth AM, Strano AJ, Chandra R, et al. Disseminated nosematosis in an immunologically compromised infant. Arch Pathol 1973;95:145–150
4. Ashton N, Wirasinha PA. Encephalitozoonosis (nosematosis) of the cornea. Br J Ophthalmol 1973;57:669–674
5. Pinnolis M, Egbert PR, Font RL, Winter FC. Nosematosis of the cornea. Arch Ophthalmol 1981;99:1044–1047
6. Bergquist NR, Stintzing G, Smedman L, et al. Diagnosis of encephalitozoonosis in man by serological tests. Br Med J 1984;288:902
7. Ledford DK, Overman MD, Gonzalvo A, et al. Microsporidiosis myositis in a patient with acquired immunodeficiency syndrome. Ann Intern Med 1985;102:628–630
8. Davis RM, Font RL, Keisler MS, Shadduck DVM. Corneal microsporidiosis. A case report including ultrastructural observations. Ophthalmology 1990;97:953–957
9. Bryan R, Cali A, Owen RL, Spencer HC. Microsporidia: newly recognized opportunistic pathogens in patients with AIDS. In: Sun T, ed. Progress in clinical parasitology. New York: Norton, 1990:1–26
10. Centers for Disease Control. Microsporidian keratoconjunctivitis in patients with AIDS. MMWR 1990;39:188–189
11. Terada S, Reddy R, Jeffers LJ, et al. Microsporidian hepatitis in the acquired immunodeficiency syndrome. Ann Intern Med 1987;107(1):61–62

12. Zender HE, Arrigoni E, Eckert J, Kapanci Y. A case of *Encephalitozoon cuniculi* peritonitis in a patient with AIDS. Am J Clin Pathol 1989;92:352–356
13. Lowder CY, Meisler DM, McMahon JT, et al. Microsporidia infection of the cornea in an HIV-positive man. Am J Ophthalmol 1990;109:242–244
14. Friedberg DN, Stenson SM, Orenstein JM, et al. Microsporidial keratoconjunctivitis in the acquired immunodeficiency syndrome. Arch Ophthalmol 1990;108:504–508
15. Yee RW, Fermin OT, Martinez J, et al. Resolution of microsporidial epithelial keratopathy in a patient with AIDS. Ophthalmology 1991;98:198–201
16. Metcalfe TW, Doran RM, Rowlands PL, et al. Microsporidial keratoconjunctivitis in a patient with AIDS. Br J Ophthalmol 1992;76(3):177–178
17. Canning EU, Lom J. The microsporidia of vertebrates. London: Academic, 1986
18. Shadduck JA, Meccoli RA, Davis R, Font RL. Isolation of a microsporidian from a human patient. J Infect Dis 1990;162:773–776
19. Didier ES, Shadduck JA, Didier PJ, et al. Studies on ocular microsporidia. J Protozool 1991;38:635–638
20. Cali A, Meisler DM, Lowder CY, et al. Corneal microsporidioses: characterization and identification. J Protozool 1991;38:215S–217S

Rapid Diagnostic Tests for Infectious Ocular Disease

Y. Jerold Gordon, M.D.

■ Clinical Need

Despite the continuing technological advances in developing and developed nations throughout the world, ocular infection remains a leading cause of ocular blindness and morbidity at the close of the twentieth century. Trachoma, measles, and bacterial corneal ulcers remain the scourge of Third World countries, whereas herpes simplex virus (HSV), contact lens–related bacterial corneal ulcers, postoperative endophthalmitis and, most recently, *Acanthamoeba* keratitis are the leading infectious causes of visual loss in the industrialized world. The need for rapid and accurate diagnosis of microbial infection of the eye remains as important today as it has been in the past.

Rapid, accurate diagnosis of ocular infection and the prompt initiation of appropriate therapy is especially important and sight-saving in *Pseudomonas* cornea ulcer, herpetic dendritic keratitis, fungal keratitis, bacterial endophthalmitis, and *Acanthamoeba* keratitis. Delay in distinguishing among many ocular microbial pathogens is not only sight-threatening in these conditions but also involves significant medicolegal liability for the ophthalmologist practicing in the United States today.

Furthermore, the cost and waste associated with improper diagnosis and attendant inappropriate use of antibiotics and antiviral agents, unnecessary office visits, and costly hospitalizations will be more difficult to justify in a future that undoubtedly includes greater physician scrutiny and monitoring under some systems of managed care. The goal to develop more rapid, accurate, and sensitive diagnostic tests for ocular pathogens is therefore appropriate today and will be energetically pursued in the near future.

■ Definition of a Rapid Diagnostic Test

In an ideal world, a rapid diagnostic test for the determination of ocular pathogens would be one whose result is available *before* the patient leaves the doctor's office, thereby allowing for the prompt initiation of proper therapy. I arbitrarily define *rapid* as less than 1 hour. Additional features of this ideal test would include excellent sensitivity and specificity, low cost, long-term shelf life, ease of performance by office staff, and no need for expensive equipment or hazardous reagents.

■ Central Laboratory Versus Office-Based Tests

Currently, all diagnostic tests for infectious ocular pathogens can be divided according to the site at which they are performed. The relative advantages and disadvantages of each will be reviewed. Traditionally, a central laboratory offers a place where all diagnostic tests (excluding the clinical examination) can be performed. The advantages include appropriate experience, expertise, equipment, and personnel. Technical sophistication is usually not an issue. However, there are also serious disadvantages. To use a central laboratory, either the patient must go there (problems of additional patient expense and inconvenience) or the sample must be delivered to it (problems of sample preservation, delivery, and the possibility of loss, breakage, or errors in handling). Both of these options preclude meeting the terms of an ideal rapid test due to the time required, the location of the patient, or both.

In contrast, office-based tests offer the theoretical advantages of meeting the terms of the proposed ideal rapid diagnostic test. However, significant disadvantages include cost, limited shelf life of kits, limited level of test sophistication, limited number of patients requiring tests, time of performance, need for trained personnel or expensive equipment (or both), and need to provide for storage and disposal of hazardous chemicals or biological wastes. Cost-effectiveness, the possible need for state licensure (depending on the specific test) and, most recently, possible conflict of interest in doctor-owned laboratories all contribute to the problems of office-based testing.

■ Current Diagnosis of Ocular Pathogens

Rapid Tests (< 1 hour)

The Table summarizes my view of the current state of testing for ocular pathogens. It includes the most common ocular pathogens that produce external disease—bacteria, viruses, fungi, chlamydiae, and *Acanthamoeba* species—and a subjective evaluation (on a scale from 1 to 4) of the value of each test in providing a reliable and accurate diagnosis. From the point of view of a busy clinician, there are very few tests that can be defined as rapid. The clinical examination, which includes history, external eye examination, and slit-lamp evaluation, has traditionally been an excellent way to diagnose ocular infection accurately. Typical cases of dendritic keratitis are invariably due to HSV [1]. A purulent conjunctivitis is usually bacterial in nature and self-limiting. Conjunctivitis is rarely a significant threat to vision, except for neonatal infection due to gonococci or streptococci that may proceed to perforation. In contrast to conjunctivitis, corneal ulceration is always serious as it is potentially vision-threatening. The failure to diagnose correctly and to treat an early *Pseudomonas* corneal ulcer can be disastrous because of the rapidity of corneal melting and perforation. Corneal ulcers due to gram-positive bacteria (*Pneumococcus* or *Staphylococcus* species) are rarely rapidly destructive, but the likely outcome of some scarring makes early treatment desirable to minimize vision loss.

Although the clinical examination may be valuable in distinguishing among different pathogens when clinical presentations are typical or pathognomonic, atypical or nonspecific findings can make the clinician's job difficult. For example, the differential diagnosis of corneal ulcer associated with localized stromal inflammation and iridocyclitis should include bacterial, herpetic, fungal, and *Acanthamoeba* ulcers, and the correct diagnosis requires additional diagnostic testing (see the Figure).

An important rapid office-based test that meets all the requirements of an ideal test and is currently available is microscopical examination of a stained smear of corneal or conjunctival specimens. A corneal scraping (see the table) demonstrates that the correct diagnosis of bacterial, fungal, and *Acanthamoeba* corneal ulcers can be reliably achieved. A Gram stain takes 5 minutes and a Giemsa stain 45 minutes to perform. These tests require minimal space, few chemical reagents, a microscope, and little experience to interpret properly. I believe that this valuable technique is currently underutilized and could better serve the busy clinician if it were used in more practices.

Intermediate Diagnostic Tests (1–6 Hours)

The next category of diagnostic tests is generally intermediate in terms of the time required for their performance (1–6 hours). These tests are immunological in nature and detect unique antigens of the ocular pathogens in question. The enzyme immunoassay (EIA) and enzyme-linked immunosorbent assay (ELISA) are the most common types, are usually available in kit form, are simple to perform, and have easy-to-interpret colorimetric end points. For the diagnosis of HSV, we and others have found the Herpcheck test (DuPont, Wilmington, DE) to have 100% sensitivity and 100% specificity for direct ocular specimens [2, 3]. However, this test is somewhat costly and takes 5 hours to perform. In contrast, Kodak

Diagnosis of Ocular Pathogens

Diagnostic test	Site	Bacteria	Virus	Fungus	*Chlamydia* Sp.	*Acanthamoeba* Sp.
Rapid (<1 hour)						
Clinical examination (10 min)	O	Purulent conjunctivitis (4)	Follicular conjunctivitis (adenovirus) (4)	Corneal ulcer (2)	Follicular conjunctivitis (2)	Contact lens wear (3)
					Pannus (3)	Stromal ring (3)
						Nerve infiltrates (4)
		Corneal ulcer (3)	HSV dendrite (4)			
Smear						
Gram stain (5 min)	O, CL	Bacteria (4)	Multinucleate giant cells (3)	Hyphae (4)	Polymorphonuclear leukocytes, lymphocytes (2)	Trophozoites (4)
Giemsa stain (45 min)		Polymorphonuclear leukocytes (3)		Yeasts (4)	Inclusions (4)	Cysts (4)
Intermediate (1–6 hours)						
Immunological tests (EIA, ELISA)	O, CL	NA	HSV Herpcheck (4) Surecell (2) ADV—Adenoclone (3)	NA	Chlamydiazyme (3) Mikrotrak (2)	NA

Serological workup	CL	*Borrelia burgdorferi* (4) (Lyme disease)	Epstein-Barr virus (infectious mononucleosis) (4)	Not useful	IgG titers (2)	NA
Late (>24 hours)						
Culture	CL	Identification 2 days (4) Sensitivity 3 days (4)	1–7 days (4)	1–7 days (4)	2 days, McCoy cells (2)	1–4 days (4)
*PCR**	CL	*Streptococcus pneumonia* *Hemophilus influenza* *Mycobacterium tuberculosis* *B. burgdorferi*	HSV CMV HIV EBV HPV	NA	*C. trachomatis*	NA
*Dot-blot**	CL ?O	*Legionella* sp.	NA	NA	NA	NA

Numbers in parentheses indicate rating of the test on a scale of 1 (poor) to 4 (diagnostic).

O = office-based; *CL* = central laboratory; *EIA* = enzyme immunoassay; *ELISA* = enzyme-linked immunosorbent assay; *PCR* = polymerase chain reaction; *NA* = not available; *HSV* = herpes simplex virus; *CMV* = cytomegalovirus; *HIV* = human immunodeficiency virus; *EBV* = Epstein-Barr virus; *HPV* = hepatitis virus.

*Molecular tests that detect unique RNA and DNA sequences.

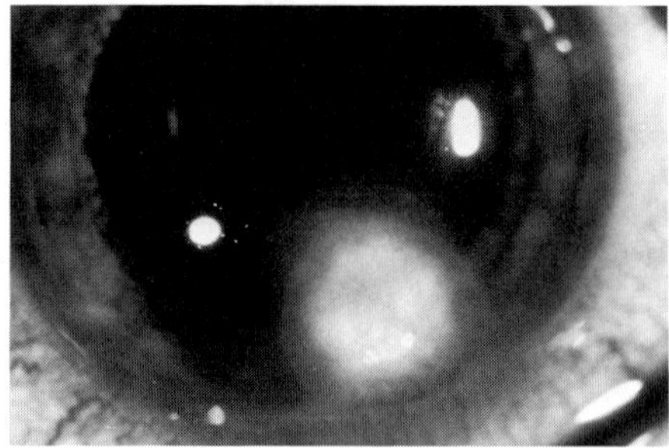

Differential diagnosis of corneal ulcer with stromal inflammation and iridocyclitis includes bacteria, herpes simplex virus, fungi, and Acanthamoeba *organisms. This ulcer was due to a* Candida *species.*

Surecell (Eastman Kodak Company, Rochester, NY) takes 15 minutes to perform, but the 27% sensitivity and 80% specificity (n = 22) that we reported [4] was less promising than preliminary data reported by Torres and colleagues [5] (70% sensitivity, 100% specificity, n = 10).

The rapid diagnosis of adenoviral keratoconjunctivitis from direct ocular specimens was assessed by comparing the Adenoclone Test (Cambridge Bioscience, Worcester, MA) to immunofiltration (V & P Scientific, San Diego, CA) [6]. For the Adenoclone Test (EIA), we found a sensitivity of 81% and a specificity of 100% for specimens taken within 1 week of the onset of clinical symptoms (n = 62), as compared to 0% when cultures were taken after 7 days (n = 13). Immunofiltration (capture of antigen on a filter using a suction manifold) was even more successful: In specimens obtained within 1 week of symptom onset, sensitivity was 79% and specificity was 100% (n = 62), whereas in specimens taken after 1 week, sensitivity was 46% and specificity was 100% (n = 13).

In the laboratory diagnosis of adult chlamydial conjunctivitis, three diagnostic tests were compared using specimens taken from 76 patients [7]. Growth of the agent *Chlamydia trachomatis* in McCoy cell culture served as the standard to evaluate Chlamydiazyme (Abbott Laboratories, North Chicago, IL), a 3-hour EIA; Mikrotrak (Syva, Palo Alto, CA), a 45-minute direct fluorescent antibody test (DFA); and Giemsa cytology (45 minutes). Overall, Chlamydiazyme proved to be the most accurate test (sensitivity 71%, specificity 97%) when compared to DFA (sensitivity 57%, specificity 81%) and Giemsa cytology (sensitivity 71%, specificity 67%).

The use of patient serological workup (measuring increasing specific serum antibodies titers) for the diagnosis of ocular infections is not rapid but has proved useful in diagnosing Lyme disease, Epstein-Barr keratitis, and chlamydial infections [8].

Late Diagnostic Tests (> 24 Hours)

The gold standard for the diagnosis of ocular pathogens has always been growing the microorganisms in cell culture. Although this technique is definitive, it is not office-based and requires a central laboratory. Cell culture methods are also not rapid, because time must be allowed for growth of the microorganism. Bacteria require 1 to 2 days for identification and another 1 to 2 days for determination of antibiotic sensitivities. Depending on serotype or isolate and inoculum, HSV and adenovirus take from 1 to 7 days to demonstrate cytopathic effect (cpe) in cell culture, and then this must be confirmed by EIA. Fungi and *Acanthamoeba* require 1 to 7 days to grow in specialized culture plates, and *Chlamydia* is relatively difficult to grow in McCoy cells. Finally, cell culture has the additional disadvantage of exposing health personnel to potentially dangerous infectious agents (hepatitis B, human immunodeficiency virus [HIV], and HSV).

■ Future Diagnostic Tests

Polymerase Chain Reaction

The diagnostic tests of the future will be safe, rapid, highly accurate, and versatile. Application of the laboratory tools of molecular biology to clinical diagnostics is at hand. Currently, these tests are undergoing development and will revolutionize the field. The polymerase chain reaction (PCR) is the prototypical technique and will be described in some detail.

PCR is based on using specific oligonucleotide probes to detect unique sequences of DNA or RNA following amplification of the target sequences in vitro [9]. There are many theoretical and practical advantages to PCR as a diagnostic tool. The versatility of the method allows it to be applied theoretically to all microorganisms, as well as for the diagnosis of genetic diseases. The outstanding specificity is based on careful selection of specific probes. The extraordinary sensitivity of the method is attributable to an amplification process (through repeated cycling) that allows for magnification of the target sequences up to 1 million times. After PCR, the proverbial 2-inch needle in a haystack would be 34 miles long! Other advantages of PCR include the safety of working with inactive DNA or RNA rather than the potentially dangerous infectious forms of the microorganisms (e.g., HIV, hepatitis B, HSV) and its usefulness in detecting slow-growing or poorly growing agents (e.g., *Chlamydia*) [10].

Despite its many advantages, there are also significant disadvantages to the present state of PCR technology. The current end points as a research tool are too cumbersome, time-consuming, and impractical for clinical diagnostic usage. These end points include fluorescent bands on an ethidium bromide gel (5 hours) and radioactive bands on a Southern blot (2 days). Because it requires expensive equipment, highly skilled laboratory personnel, extensive physical space, and radioactive materials, PCR technology is too expensive and impractical for office use.

The technique is plagued by false-positive results from errant DNA, and extraordinary precautions must be taken to avoid this outcome in a clinical situation. Sampling error may also be a problem in the detection of very rare sequences, as the volume of the sample to be tested is so small (20 µl). Our laboratory has applied PCR to clinical ocular swabs for the detection of HSV using thymidine kinase probes. Comparing results from ethidium bromide gels to Southern blots, we determined that as sensitivity increased from 86% (19/22) to 95% (20/21), specificity declined from 85% (17/20) to 65% (13/20). These results suggest that it will be very important clinically to optimize conditions to obtain the highest sensitivity without sacrificing specificity [2].

At the present time, PCR technology is being modified and developed for practical application in a clinical laboratory setting. The original technology was developed by Cetus Corporation, and Perkin-Elmer manufactured the PCR machines. Recently, Hoffmann-La Roche has acquired the rights to commercialize the technology. Following approval by the U.S. Food and Drug Administration, diagnostic tests for AIDS, Lyme disease, and *Chlamydia* infection will be among the first clinical applications of PCR [11].

Dot-Blot Test

Dot-blot testing has already employed PCR technology for the rapid detection of *Legionella pneumophila*, a bacterial contaminant of water responsible for the often fatal Legionnaire's disease. The EnviroAmp Legionella Kit, as developed by Perkin-Elmer Cetus, uses a reverse dot-blot method with a colorimetric end point (blue dots) that provides results in 4 hours [12].

■ Summary

There is a current and ongoing need for the rapid, accurate diagnosis of ocular infection and the prompt initiation of appropriate therapy to prevent visual loss, maximize use of health care resources, and reduce physicians' medicolegal liability. For the busy clinician, an ideal rapid diagnostic test to determine ocular pathogens would be one whose result is available *before* the patient leaves the doctor's office, so that optimal treatment can be promptly instituted. Today, the major rapid diagnostic tests available to the busy clinician are the clinical examination and the stained microscopical smear of conjunctival and corneal specimens. The latter technique is grossly underutilized and would contribute significantly to improved accuracy in early diagnosis of ocular infections. In the near future, improved enzyme immunoassays and simplified PCR kits will provide for highly sensitive and specific diagnostic capabilities for detecting ocular pathogens in the laboratory and, possibly, office settings.

The author has no financial interest in any of the products described and received no compensation for testing the products.

This study was supported in part by grants from the National Institutes of Health (NEI EY05232, EY08227), Bethesda, MD; The Charles T. Campbell Foundation, Pittsburgh, PA; Research to Prevent Blindness, Inc., New York, NY; and the Eye and Ear Institute of Pittsburgh.

■ References

1. Kowalski RP, Gordon YJ. Evaluation of immunologic tests for the detection of ocular herpes simplex virus. Ophthalmology 1989;96:1583–1586
2. Kowalski RP, Romanowski EG, Araullo-Cruz T, Gordon YJ. Immunoassay, PCR of slit-lamp diagnosis: which is superior for detecting ocular HSV disease? Invest Ophthalmol Vis Sci 1991;32(suppl):805
3. Dunkel EC, Pavan-Langston D, Fitzpatrick K, Culor G. Rapid detection of herpes simplex virus (HSV) antigen in human ocular infections. Curr Eye Res 1988; 7:661–666
4. Kowalski RP, Portnoy SL, Karenchak LM, Arffa R. The evaluation of the Kodak Surecell test for the detection of ocular herpes simplex virus. Am J Ophthalmol 1991;112:214–215
5. Torres MA, Asbell PA, Kamenar T, et al. Rapid diagnosis of herpes simplex ocular infections. Invest Ophthalmol Vis Sci 1990;31(suppl):221
6. Kowalski RP, Gordon YJ. Comparison of direct rapid tests for the detection of adenovirus antigen in routine conjunctival specimens. Ophthalmology 1989;96: 1106–1109
7. Sheppard JD, Kowalski RP, Meyer MP, et al. Immunodiagnosis of adult chlamydial conjunctivitis. Ophthalmology 1988;95:434–443
8. Springer DS, Kowalski RP, Wiley LA, et al. The value of serum IgG titers in diagnosing adult chlamydial keratoconjunctivitis (ACK). Invest Ophthalmol Vis Sci 1988;29(suppl):38
9. Rodu B. The polymerase chain reaction: the revolution within. Am J Med Sci 1990;299:210–216
10. Ostergaard L, Birkelund S, Christiansen G. Use of the polymerase chain reaction for detection of *Chlamydia trachomatis*. J Clin Microbiol 1990;28:1254–1260
11. Gibbons A. Hoffmann-La Roche's PCR push. Science 9 Aug 1991;253:627
12. Erdman V. Perkin-Elmer Cetus pioneers PCR-based environmental test kits: EnviroAMP *Legionella* kit. Perkin-Elmer Instrument News 1992;2:4

Role of the Fluoroquinolones in Ophthalmology

Olivia N. Serdarevic, M.D.

The fluoroquinolone antibiotics represent a new therapeutic option in the treatment of ocular disease. Although the prototype agent, nalidixic acid, has been available for systemic use since 1962 [1], the broader-spectrum fluoroquinolones were introduced for oral use in the early 1980s and for parenteral and topical ophthalmic use in the mid-1980s. The fluoroquinolones are structural analogs of nalidixic acid with a fluorine group in position 6 to increase antimicrobial potency and a piperazine ring in position 7 to enhance the antimicrobial spectrum (Figure). The structural differences (see the Figure) among the fluoroquinolones available for topical ophthalmic use (ofloxacin, norfloxacin, and ciprofloxacin) alter their potency and pharmacokinetic profiles [2]. The addition of a methyl group to the piperazine ring, as in ofloxacin, increases lipophilicity and, thereby, enhances absorption and penetration in tissues. The ring connecting position 1 to position 8 of the quinolone nucleus increases the solubility of ofloxacin as compared to norfloxacin and ciprofloxacin. A cyclopropyl group at position 1, as in ciprofloxacin, increases activity against *Pseudomonas aeruginosa* and Enterobacteriaceae.

Mode of Action

All the fluoroquinolones are bactericidal and interfere with DNA gyrase, a type 2 topoisomerase [3]. DNA gyrase catalyzes DNA supercoiling. It also is involved in DNA replication, transcription, recombination, and repair. The fluoroquinolones show high specificity for bacterial DNA gyrase, since mammalian cells possess a structurally different DNA gyrase that has no supercoiling activity. These antimicrobials bind to DNA gyrase and prevent DNA gyrase from resealing DNA strands. In addition to their bactericidal action, the fluoroquinolones exhibit a postantibiotic effect and inhibit bacterial growth for 2 to 6 hours [4].

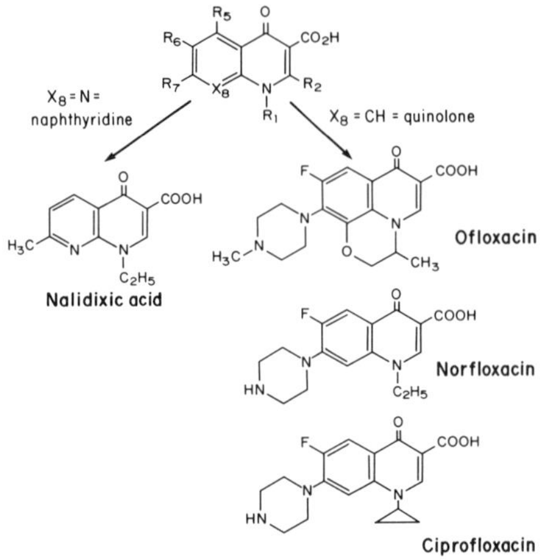

The chemical structure of the fluoroquinolones is analogous to that of nalidixic acid. A fluorine group in position 6 enhances antimicrobial potency, and a piperazine ring in position 7 broadens the antimicrobial spectrum.

Some of the fluoroquinolones have additional mechanisms that are not completely understood but that, unlike the DNA gyrase mechanism, function in the absence of cell multiplication and protein synthesis [5]. These mechanisms may be related to alterations of the cell membrane and are drug- and bacteria-specific. Of the three ophthalmic preparations, only ofloxacin and ciprofloxacin possess these mechanisms against *Escherichia coli* and only ofloxacin possesses them against staphylococci.

■ Antimicrobial Activity

The fluoroquinolones offer the potential for improved antimicrobial therapy because of their potency and broad spectrum of activity. Although in vitro activity does not always correlate with in vivo efficacy, in vitro data against ocular pathogens are, nevertheless, indicators of probable clinical efficacy. The fluoroquinolones demonstrate low minimum inhibitory concentrations (MICs) against both gram-positive and gram-negative bacteria. The Table is a compilation of data from several published studies [6–8] and lists the MICs against 90% of the common ocular isolates tested.

Ofloxacin and ciprofloxacin are more potent than the aminoglycosides and chloramphenicol against gram-positive bacteria. Other fluoroquinolones that are not yet available commercially, such as tosufloxacin, have even lower MICs—in the range of 0.12 to 0.25 µg/ml [9]—and are more potent against gram-positive cocci. Norfloxacin demonstrates high MICs against streptococci and, therefore, should not be used to treat streptococcal infections. In recent studies, ofloxacin demonstrated better activity than ciprofloxacin in vitro against streptococci. Using standardized broth dilution susceptibility methods, Veights and colleagues [10] found 91% of ocular strains of *Streptococcus pneumoniae* susceptible to ofloxacin but only 65%

In Vitro Antibacterial Activity of Selected Agents Against Ocular Isolates

Organism	Minimum Inhibitory Concentration 90 (μg/ml)					
	Ofloxacin	Norfloxacin	Ciprofloxacin	Tobramycin	Gentamicin	Chloramphenicol
Staphylococcus aureus	0.5	1.0–2.0	0.6	1.0–2.0	0.5–1.0	4.0–16
Staphylococcus epidermidis	0.5	2.0	0.5	64	32	32
Streptococcus pneumoniae	2.0	14.4–32	2.0	16–32	7.0–32	4.0
Pseudomonas aeruginosa	4.0	1.0–4.0	0.7	1.0–4.4	2.0–8.0	64–128
Hemophilus influenzae	4.0	1.0–16	0.03–0.06	2.0	1.0–4.0	1.0–20

Source: Compiled from published data [6–8].

of the strains susceptible to ciprofloxacin. Kowalski and collaborators [unpublished data, 1991] demonstrated susceptibility of 100% of the strains of *S. pneumoniae* and 92% of the strains of alpha-hemolytic streptococci to ofloxacin compared with susceptibility of 69% and 25% of the strains, respectively, to ciprofloxacin. Enterococci are inhibited by ofloxacin and ciprofloxacin but not by norfloxacin. The fluoroquinolones, especially ofloxacin and ciprofloxacin, provide good coverage against spore-forming bacilli such as *Bacillus* species and non-spore-forming bacilli such as *Corynebacterium* species.

Ciprofloxacin is the most potent of the fluoroquinolones available for ophthalmic use against gram-negative bacteria, but all compare favorably with the aminoglycosides. The fluoroquinolones inhibit gram-negative diplococci, rods, diplobacilli, and coccobacilli.

Fluoroquinolone action against anaerobes is variable. *Propionibacterium acnes* usually is sensitive, but many *Clostridium* and *Bacteroides* species are not inhibited by available fluoroquinolones. Acid-fast bacteria are variably inhibited by fluoroquinolones. Some mycobacteria are susceptible, but *Nocardia* species are resistant. Although norfloxacin provides inadequate coverage against chlamydial species, ciprofloxacin and particularly ofloxacin inhibit these organisms.

The fluoroquinolones are bactericidal, since the minimal bactericidal concentrations (MBCs) are only one to two times the MIC for most isolates [11].

■ Pharmacokinetics

Effective drug concentrations must be achieved and maintained at infection sites in order to obtain optimal therapeutic response. In a randomized, double-masked clinical trial, Schwob and colleagues [12] calculated the duration that tear concentrations exceeded MICs [6] for common ocular pathogens following administration of 0.3% topical ofloxacin solution or 0.3% tobramycin solution four times daily for 12 doses. Both ofloxacin and tobramycin maintained effective tear concentrations for more than 4 hours for *P. aeruginosa* and *Hemophilus influenzae*. However, antibiotic levels effective against gram-positive bacteria were maintained in the tear film much longer with ofloxacin than with tobramycin. Tear ofloxacin levels exceeded MICs for *Staphylococcus epidermidis* for more than 16 hours and for *S. pneumoniae* for more than 8 hours, whereas tear tobramycin levels were below effective levels for these organisms in 15 to 30 minutes. These data suggest that dosing of fluoroquinolone ophthalmic solutions may not be required as frequently as that of aminoglycoside solutions.

In vivo activity of the fluoroquinolones does not always correlate with in vitro activity since drug absorption, tissue penetration, and metabolism will affect the latter. The corneal epithelium is a major barrier for many ocular medications. The enhanced lipophilicity of some of the fluoroquinolones, such as ofloxacin, pefloxacin, and temafloxacin, facilitates penetration through intact corneal epithelium and prolongs drug half-life [2]. Animal studies [13] and clinical trials [WB Jackson, unpublished data, 1992] have demonstrated the ability of ofloxacin to penetrate intact corneal epithelium better than tobramycin and to achieve higher concentrations in the aqueous humor. All three fluoroquinolones available as 0.3% ophthalmic solutions achieve corneal and conjunctival concentrations substantially above the MICs for most pathogens. There have been very few studies comparing ocular penetration and diffusion of different fluoroquinolones. Reidy and collaborators [14] compared drug aqueous humor levels 1 hour after administering 0.75% ciprofloxacin drops or 1% norfloxacin drops every 15 minutes for four doses and every 30 minutes for 3 hours in rabbit corneas with *Pseudomonas* keratitis. The mean aqueous concentration of the ciprofloxacin-treated eyes was significantly higher (30.5 μg/ml $\pm$ 2.5 SEM) than that of the norfloxacin-treated eyes (7.5 μg/ml $\pm$ 0.23 SEM) ($p <$ .0001). Studies of aqueous humor penetration through intact epithelium after topical application in human eyes indicate that concentrations exceeding the MICs of most bacteria are obtained with ciprofloxacin [15] and ofloxacin [WB Jackson, unpublished data, 1992] but not with norfloxacin [16, 17]. Removal of the corneal epithelial barrier greatly enhances penetration of topical fluoroquinolones [13] into anterior segment tissue, but vitreal concentrations are minimal and below therapeutic levels. Topical ophthalmic treatment yields far lower serum levels than standard oral regimens [18, 19]. Borrmann and co-workers [18] measured the maximum serum concentration of ofloxacin after 10 days of topical administration as being more than 1,000 times lower than the maximum serum concentration after a single 200- to 300-mg oral dose of ofloxacin. Leibowitz [19] reported that the mean peak ciprofloxacin plasma level obtained after 7-day topical dosing for treatment of conjunctivitis or keratitis was approximately 450 times less than that measured after a single 250-mg oral dose of ciprofloxacin.

Corneal collagen shields have been used as drug delivery devices. Studies have demonstrated that collagen shields can be saturated with antibiotics that are released as the shields dissolve [20]. There are no published reports to date describing the pharmacokinetics of fluoroquinolone delivery from collagen shields.

Very few studies have investigated ocular fluoroquinolone levels after subconjunctival injection. The results of animal studies suggest that therapeutic aqueous but not vitreous levels can be achieved at 1 hour after subconjunctival injections of ciprofloxacin at nontoxic concentrations of 6 to 12 mg/ml [21].

Most recent studies of vitreal fluoroquinolone levels following intravitreal injections have evaluated ciprofloxacin. At 1 hour after a 100-µg intravitreal injection of ciprofloxacin in rabbit eyes, peak vitreal levels were obtained [22], and drug levels exceeding MICs were obtained even 48 hours after injection [23]. However, vitreal ciprofloxacin levels after intravitreal injection fall below MIC levels for gram-positive bacteria much faster in vitrectomized animals [24], suggesting the need for multiple dosing to maintain bactericidal levels.

The fluoroquinolones are well absorbed orally. After a dose of 400 mg, ofloxacin and pefloxacin achieve higher peak serum doses and have longer serum half-lives than ciprofloxacin and norfloxacin [25]. The peak aqueous humor concentrations of ofloxacin and pefloxacin after systemic administration are higher than those of ciprofloxacin [26–31] and exceed MICs for both gram-positive and gram-negative bacteria. El Baba and associates [32] reported that vitreous levels of ciprofloxacin were clinically insignificant for up to almost 5 hours after oral administration of a 750-mg dose prior to vitreous surgery. Then, from approximately 5 hours to more than 16 hours afterward, ciprofloxacin vitreous levels exceeded the MICs for some bacteria but not for *Staphylococcus aureus* and *Pseudomonas* species. Higher intravitreal ciprofloxacin levels were obtained after two oral doses given 12 hours apart [33].

■ Development of Resistance

Plasmidborne resistance is considered the most significant resistance problem leading to therapeutic failure with conventional antibiotics. The fluoroquinolones have been exempt from plasmid-transferred resistance, but resistance can occur through chromosomal mutations. Spontaneous mutations occur at frequencies in the range of 1×10^8 to 1×10^{12}. However, because of the widespread systemic use of ciprofloxacin in the United States, there have been reports of increasing resistance in staphylococcal infections [34]. Frequent systemic use of pefloxacin and ofloxacin in Europe has led to the emergence of resistant strains of *Pseudomonas* [JP Adenis, F Denis, personal communication, 1992]. Most cases of bacterial resistance to fluoroquinolones, however, involve nosocomial infections and long-term monotherapy. Although cross-resistance for selected mutants to fluoroquinolones has been observed, the potential for cross-resistance with other antibiotics is low [35], occurring to date mainly in methicillin-resistant staphylococci.

In vitro studies of the frequency and stability of spontaneous resistant mutants can be useful in predicting clinical failure related to the selection of strains with decreased susceptibility to specific antibiotic therapy. Piddock and Wise [35] demonstrated that *S. pneumoniae* yielded mutants to twice the MIC of ofloxacin, norfloxacin, and ciprofloxacin at a frequency associated with a mutation at a single gene. However, only 6% of selected mutants had a twofold decrease in susceptibility to ofloxacin, whereas 25% of norfloxacin-selected mutants and 100% of ciprofloxacin-selected mutants had a twofold decrease. At four times the MIC of ofloxacin and ciprofloxacin, no resistant mutants were detected, but 50% of norfloxacin-selected mutants demonstrated more than a fourfold increase in MIC. Moreover, 83% of the mutants selected with ofloxacin were nonviable, whereas 100% of the ciprofloxacin mutants and 95% of the norfloxacin mutants were viable. Therapeutic failure is associated with viable resistant mutants. Ofloxacin-resistant mutants are reported to be very unstable and readily revert to ofloxacin sensitivity [36]. Clinical experience will reveal whether ofloxacin-resistant mutants truly have a reduced probability of being fully competent pathogens compared to mutants resistant to norfloxacin, ciprofloxacin, and nonfluoroquinolone antibiotics.

■ Adverse Effects

For antibiotics to be clinically useful, they should be effective with minimal adverse effects. Topical fluoroquinolones are generally well tolerated [37–41] and compare favorably with other topical antibiotics. The incidence of ocular adverse effects reported in clinical trials evaluating the efficacy of fluoroquinolones in the treatment of external eye infections and keratitis ranges from 0.8% in 1,284 patients treated with ofloxacin topical therapy [MJ Branin, personal communication, 1992] to 9.7% in 1,520 patients treated with ciprofloxacin topical therapy [19]. Ocular irritation and discomfort were the most frequently cited adverse reactions. The decreased frequency of ocular irritation noted during ofloxacin therapy may be related to differences in the formulations of the commercially available fluoroquinolone solutions. Ciprofloxacin and norfloxacin topical solutions are buffered and contain both benzalkonium chloride (BAK) and edetate disodium (EDTA), whereas ofloxacin solution is not buffered and contains BAK but not EDTA. Both BAK and EDTA have been documented to be toxic to the corneal epithelium when applied very frequently [42, 43]. Formulations that contain both of these chemical preservatives have been reported to be more damaging to corneal cells than formulations containing only one [44]. The corneal epithelial cytotoxicity of unpreserved fluoroquinolones was evaluated in vitro by Cutarelli and colleagues [45] and found to be minimal at clinical concentrations compared to that of the aminoglycosides and cephalosporins. Although ciprofloxacin demonstrated even less epithelial toxicity than ofloxacin and norfloxacin in that study, it has been found to cause white crystalline precipitation on the surface of 16.6% of corneal ulcers in clinical studies [19]. These precipitates sometimes interfere with reepithelialization unless removed by irrigation or mechanically [ON Serdarevic, unpublished data, 1992]. The increased solubility at pH 7 of ofloxacin compared to ciprofloxacin may account for the absence of reports of ofloxacin precipitation. Apart from a taste abnormality that has been experienced by 5.0% of patients during topical ciprofloxacin treatment in clinical trials [19, 40], nonocular side effects (including nausea and headache) were reported after topical fluoroquinolone therapy at an incidence of less than 1.0% [37–41].

Conjunctival precipitates have been observed in animal studies after subconjunctival ciprofloxacin injections of 6 to 40 mg [21]. Katz and associates [21] also noted marked conjunctival edema with areas of ischemic necrosis and hemorrhage in rabbit eyes receiving subconjunctival doses greater than 12 mg/ml.

The intraocular safety of intravitreal fluoroquinolone administration also has been studied only in animal models to date. No acute ocular toxicity was detected in phakic or aphakic vitrectomized rabbits after intravitreal instillation of 100 μg ciprofloxacin hydrochloride that achieved an inhibitory quotient of 220 to 250 and, thereby, allowed a threefold safety margin [46]. Retinal toxicity was evaluated by electroretinography, light microscopy, and transmission electron microscopy (TEM). TEM was found to be the most sensitive method for determining retinal toxicity and revealed outer retinal damage at intravitreal doses of 250 μg or more. Dose-dependent corneal decompensation that was demonstrated by increased corneal thickness with associated bullous keratopathy occurred in aphakic vitrectomized eyes after intravitreal ciprofloxacin injections of greater than 100 μg. In the same study, Stevens and co-workers [46] observed reversible corneal decompensation in rabbits after ciprofloxacin injections of 25 μg or more into the anterior chamber and speculated that ciprofloxacin might have interfered with endothelial cell replication and pump function by inhibiting endothelial type 2 topoisomerase. The very high concentrations of fluoroquinolones achieved in the anterior chamber could inhibit not only prokaryotic DNA gyrase but also eukaryotic type 2 topoisomerases [47].

Ofloxacin, norfloxacin, ciprofloxacin, and pefloxacin have been well tolerated systemically with few reported adverse effects [48]. The most frequently reported reactions after oral and intravenous administration are gastrointestinal symptoms, including nausea, vomiting, and abdominal discomfort, in approximately 5% of patients and neurological symptoms including, most commonly, headache or dizziness and, less frequently, anxiety or depression in approximately 4% of patients. Seizures, renal failure, and hepatic failure have been reported rarely. Temafloxacin has been withdrawn from worldwide markets as a result of serious adverse reactions including severe hypoglycemia, hemolytic anemia, hepatic dysfunction, renal failure, anaphylaxis, and death. Fluoroquinolones generally are not administered systemically in children, since damage to cartilage has been observed in studies in young animals.

■ Applications in Ocular Infection

Conjunctivitis

Although many cases of acute bacterial conjunctivitis are self-limiting and resolve without antibiotic therapy, topical therapy is recommended to eradicate pathogens, prevent spread to adjacent tissues and other individuals, shorten the clinical course, and reduce the incidence of serious sequelae [49]. Hyperacute conjunctivitis caused by *Neisseria* species should be treated with systemic as well as topical antibiotics. Both gram-positive and gram-negative bacteria cause conjunctivitis, but staphylococcal species are most frequently isolated [38, 40]. *Hemophilus* species and *S. pneumoniae* often cause conjunctivitis in the pediatric age group. In patients in whom bacterial conjunctivitis is diagnosed on the basis of clinical examination, only approximately 50% of conjunctival cultures are positive [38, 40]. Although microbiological investigation should be performed routinely, the cost and delay of such investigation preclude the feasibility, in general ophthalmology practices, of obtaining cultures in all cases of nonsevere conjunctivitis and necessitate the use of broad-spectrum antibiotics. Combined antibiotic products such as those containing polymyxin B sulfate and trimethoprim sulfate or bacitracin have been developed to increase the antimicrobial coverage of commercially available antibiotics. Some of the combined products, such as those with neomycin, have been associated with an increased incidence of hypersensitivity reactions. Many ophthalmologists routinely use aminoglycosides for conjunctivitis. Erythromycin or bacitracin ointment sometimes is used in conjunction with an aminoglycoside to improve gram-positive coverage.

Initial ophthalmic clinical studies involving the fluoroquinolones evaluated their efficacy in the treatment of conjunctivitis. Placebo-controlled trials demonstrated that topical treatment with ciprofloxacin or norfloxacin significantly improved bacterial eradication and produced more rapid clinical resolution than the vehicle [40, 41]. Multicenter, randomized, double-masked clinical trials comparing 0.3% tobramycin drops with 0.3% ciprofloxacin drops [40] and 0.3% ofloxacin drops [38] demonstrated that these two fluoroquinolones were at least as effective as tobramycin in eradicating or reducing the pathogens. The fluoroquinolones eradicated 100% of the gram-negative isolates but not all of the gram-positive isolates. In vitro sensitivity testing of the culture specimens in the ofloxacin study revealed that, whereas none of the gram-negative organisms and only 0.5% of the gram-positive organisms were resistant to ofloxacin, 5.6% of the gram-negative and 14% of the gram-positive bacteria were resistant to tobramycin. Although neither study compared the fluoroquinolones directly, a larger percentage of gram-positive bacteria were not eradicated by ciprofloxacin than by ofloxacin. The severity of signs and symptoms was reduced significantly more ($p < 0.05$) with ofloxacin than with tobramycin after 3 to 5 days of treatment.

Some of the fluoroquinolones, especially ofloxacin, are very active against chlamydia. Topical ofloxacin can be used in conjunction with oral doses of 400 mg twice daily for 7 days to treat chlamydial conjunctivitis as effectively as doxycycline [9].

Although data to date suggest that topical fluoroquinolone treatment of conjunctivitis is very successful, these antibiotics should be reserved for more severe infections. Bacterial resistance to the fluoroquinolones will continue to increase most probably as a result of systemic overuse. Nevertheless, ophthalmic overuse for mild external eye infections should be avoided.

Keratitis

The failure to treat bacterial keratitis promptly and adequately can have disastrous consequences. Pathogens should be eliminated as rapidly as possible to avoid corneal damage. Although cultures and stains should be obtained in all patients, initial treatment should not be based solely on Gram stain interpretations, because they do not always correlate with culture results [50]. In the United States, staphylococcal species and *Pseudomonas* are the most frequently isolated pathogens [19, 51]. However, in the ciprofloxacin clinical trial, 39% of the ulcers were found to be polymicrobial [19]. Most corneal specialists, therefore, have advocated initial treatment with broad-spectrum coverage using fortified concentrations of an aminoglycoside and a cephalosporin or vancomycin [51]. These fortified concentrations are not available commercially and must be carefully mixed by the ophthalmologist or pharmacist every week to avoid contamination. Some of the fortified antibiotic preparations are unstable. Cefazolin demonstrates changes in pH when stored at 25°C and reduced efficacy after 7 days even when stored at 4°C [52]. Vancomycin shows significant osmolality changes over time and has a very low pH (3.61) that is in the range barely tolerated by the eye [52]. Moreover, more staphylococcal strains resistant to both cefazolin and vancomycin and more *Pseudomonas* strains resistant to the aminoglycosides are developing [53–55]. In view of these problems associated with commonly used fortified preparations, there has been great interest in topical, nonfortified fluoroquinolone therapy for bacterial keratitis.

Darrell and colleagues [56, 57] investigated the potential of fluoroquinolones for the treatment of corneal ulcers using norfloxacin. Subsequent clinical experience has demonstrated that norfloxacin inadequately covers some gram-positive organisms [9].

Recent interest has centered on ofloxacin and ciprofloxacin. Leibowitz [19] reported on the results of a multicenter prospective study comparing 0.3% ciprofloxacin to "standard" treatment for bacterial keratitis. Controls consisted of patients not enrolled in the study and patients treated for up to 1 year prior to the study. Both clinical and antibacterial efficacy were evaluated. Clinical success was defined as either a cure or improvement at the last follow-up visit. Ciprofloxacin treatment was found to have a 91.9% success rate. Standard therapy was clinically successful in 88.2% of the not-enrolled patients and in 88.3% of the historical controls. Clinical success with ciprofloxacin did not correlate in all cases with microbiological in vitro testing. *Corynebacterium* and *Staphylococcus warneri* were resistant in vitro, but ciprofloxacin treatment was successful. Several unsuccessful treatments, however, involved staphylococcal and streptococcal species that were susceptible in vitro. Based on in vitro data, ofloxacin should elicit fewer treatment failures in ulcers produced by gram-positive organisms. It is hoped that the ongoing multicenter, randomized, double-masked clinical trial comparing ofloxacin with fortified tobramycin and cefazolin will demonstrate whether single-agent therapy with ofloxacin should be the initial choice for treatment of bacterial keratitis.

The ease of administering commercially available fluoroquinolones may facilitate prompt treatment during the early stages of infection. Experimental data [15, 58] substantiated the clinically recognized importance of early antibiotic therapy during maximal bacterial replication. In cases of deep ulceration with impending or actual perforation or in cases of corneal ulceration associated with scleritis, topical fluoroquinolone therapy should be supplemented with systemic treatment. Pefloxacin and ofloxacin achieve therapeutic aqueous humor levels for most ocular pathogens without the need for intravenous medications. Additional antibiotic coverage may be required for severe infections. Currently available fluoroquinolone therapy should not be used without other antibiotic coverage in anaerobic and gram-positive aerobic infections. Newer fluoroquinolones that are being evaluated experimentally may further improve single-agent broad-spectrum therapy for corneal ulcers in the future.

Perioperative Antibiotic Prophylaxis

The use of perioperative antibiotics to prevent postoperative infection including, most importantly, endophthalmitis is still controversial [59]. The low incidence of postoperative endophthalmitis has made it difficult to identify predisposing factors and to prove the efficacy of prophylactic therapy.

Bacteria in periocular flora can be introduced into the eye during surgery. Speaker and associates [60] have demonstrated that in some cases of staphylococcal endophthalmitis, the patient's external tissues were the source of the infecting organism. However, there frequently is a lack of correlation between bacteria isolated from preoperative conjunctival and eyelid margin cultures and the causative organisms [61]. Consequently, many surgeons advocate the use of broad-spectrum antibiotics rather than preselecting antibiotics solely on the basis of preoperative culture results. Nevertheless, none of the topical antibiotics that routinely have been used preoperatively have been capable of eradicating all microbial flora in all patients.

Tamura and associates [62] evaluated the use of topical ofloxacin for preoperative antimicrobial prophylaxis in 367 patients. Ofloxacin was instilled five times daily for 2 days prior to intraocular surgery. All 92 strains isolated were found to be highly susceptible to ofloxacin, whereas 75 to 86% of them were highly sensitive to aminoglycosides and beta-lactams. Sterilization of the conjunctival sac was reported to have been achieved in almost 100% of the cases. Eyelid margins were not cultured in that study. Jackson and collaborators compared ofloxacin drops to tobramycin drops for antimicrobial prophylaxis when administered five times the night prior to and five times starting 2 hours prior to cataract extraction. Preliminary data [WB Jackson, unpublished data, 1992] revealed no significant difference between the antibiotics in terms of conjunctival and eyelid margin sterilization. Despite no demonstrable advantage of ofloxacin over tobramycin in terms of periocular flora eradication, significantly higher anterior chamber concentrations that exceeded the MICs for most ocular pathogens were achieved with ofloxacin at 1 to 3 hours after administration. Aqueous humor concentrations also were measured to be in excess of MICs after topical ofloxacin instillation in the Japanese study [62].

Although there are no published reports regarding preoperative prophylaxis after topical administration of other fluoroquinolones, ocular penetration data suggest that ciprofloxacin also would achieve therapeutic levels in the aqueous humor but that norfloxacin would not be as beneficial. A distinct disadvantage of fluoroquinolone preoperative prophylaxis would be overuse of fluoroquinolones with subsequent risk of increasing resistance and decreased efficacy during treatment of severe ocular infections.

The role of subconjunctival injections of fluoroquinolones has not been determined, but the risk-benefit ratio of postoperative subconjunctival antibiotic prophylaxis in general needs to be reconsidered [59]. Antibiotic-induced macular infarction was reported to occur after subconjunctival injections of gentamicin at the end of anterior segment surgery [63]. Since topical fluoroquinolone administration can achieve therapeutic intraocular levels even in the presence of intact corneal epithelium, subconjunctival injections can be avoided.

Oral antibiotic prophylaxis has not been widely used because of poor intraocular penetration of most antibiotics in noninflamed eyes. The fluoroquinolones, particularly pefloxacin and ofloxacin, allow much better ocular penetration and will reopen the debate of systemic prophylaxis.

Endophthalmitis

Although the incidence of endophthalmitis is low, the outcome often is devastating. Most cases of endophthalmitis occur postoperatively, but approximately 25% result from ocular trauma [64]. In a compilation of 11 studies totaling 327 cases, 65% of the isolated pathogens were gram-positive, principally *S. epidermidis,* and 24% were gram-negative [65]. Aminoglycosides and cephalosporins have been the most frequently prescribed antibiotics. However, because of relatively poor vitreal penetration and substantial systemic adverse effects, intravitreal injections routinely are administered. Retinal toxicity has been reported even after minimally therapeutic doses of gentamicin [63]. More bacteria resistant to these antibiotics are emerging.

Newer antibiotics such as imipenem, fosfomycin, and third-generation cephalosporins achieve therapeutic levels in the vitreous and have been used extensively in Europe. Orally administered fluoroquinolones, usually in conjunction with another antibiotic, also are used on a widespread basis in Europe for the treatment of endophthalmitis [JP Adenis, personal communication, 1992]. Pefloxacin and ofloxacin achieve higher peak aqueous humor and vitreal concentrations and have longer serum half-lives than ciprofloxacin and norfloxacin and, therefore, require less frequent dosing. Intravitreal therapeutic levels are maintained for shorter periods for *S. aureus* and pseudomonads than for *S. epidermidis, Bacillus* species, and Enterobacteriaceae. Because of the rapidity of bactericidal effect, it has been suggested that steroids can be started earlier after fluoroquinolone treatment than after treatment with other antibiotics [64]. Fluoroquinolones should never be used alone for endophthalmitis, since resistance to staphylococcal species and pseudomonads can develop. Oral fluoroquinolones may prove to be especially useful for antibiotic prophylaxis after ocular injury. Experimental studies [22–24] indicate that intravitreal injections of fluoroquinolones may be effective in the treatment of endophthalmitis once definitive toxicity data are acquired.

■ References

1. Lesher GY, Froelich ED, Gruet MD, et al. 1,8-Naphthyridine derivatives. A new class of chemotherapeutic agents. J Med Pharm Chem 1962;5:1063
2. Borrmann LR, Leopold IH. The potential use of quinolones in future ocular antimicrobial therapy. Am J Ophthalmol 1988;106:227–229
3. Wolfson JS, Hooper DC. The fluoroquinolones: structures, mechanisms of action and resistance, and spectra of activity in vitro. Antimicrob Agents Chemother 1985;28:581–586
4. Craig WA, Gudmundsson S. The post-antibiotic effect. In: Lorian V, ed. Antibiotics in laboratory medicine. Baltimore: Williams & Wilkins, 1986:515–536
5. Lewin CS, Smith JT. Bactericidal mechanisms of ofloxacin. J Antimicrob Chemother 1988;22:1S–8S
6. Osato MS, Jensen HG, Trousdale MD, et al. The comparative in vitro activity of ofloxacin and selected ophthalmic antimicrobial agents against ocular bacterial isolates. Am J Ophthalmol 1989;108:380–386

7. Cokingtin CD, Hyndiuk MD. Insights from experimental data on ciprofloxacin in the treatment of bacterial keratitis and ocular infections. Am J Ophthalmol 1991; 112:25S–28S

8. Goldstein EL, Citron DM, Bendon L, et al. Potential of topical norfloxacin therapy: comparative in vitro activity against clinical ocular bacterial isolates. Arch Ophthalmol 1987;105:991–994

9. Neu HC. Microbiologic aspects of fluoroquinolones. Am J Ophthalmol 1991;112: 15S–24S

10. Veights SA, Dick JD, O'Brien TP, et al. Comparative in vitro activities of fluoroquinolones vs aminoglycoside against ocular isolates. Invest Ophthalmol Vis Sci 1992;33:936

11. Reeves DS, Bywater MJ, Holt HA, White LO. In vitro studies with ciprofloxacin, a new 4-quinolone compound. J Antimicrob Chemother 1984;13:333

12. Schwob DL, Tang-Liu D, Usansky J, Gordon YJ. Comparison of the effective tear concentrations of ofloxacin versus tobramycin after multiple eyedrop administration to human eyes. Invest Ophthalmol Vis Sci 1992;33:775

13. Gritz DC, McDonnell PJ, Lee TY, et al. Topical ofloxacin in the treatment of *Pseudomonas* keratitis in a rabbit model. Cornea 1992;11:143–147

14. Reidy JJ, Hobden JA, Hill JM, et al. The efficacy of topical ciprofloxacin and norfloxacin in the treatment of experimental *Pseudomonas* keratitis. Cornea 1991; 10:25–28

15. O'Brien TP, Sawusch MR, Dick JD, Gottsch JD. Topical ciprofloxacin treatment of *Pseudomonas* keratitis in rabbits. Arch Ophthalmol 1988;106:1444–1446

16. Behrens-Baumann W. Kammerwasserkonzentration von norfloxacin nach lokaler applikation. Ophthalmologica 1991;202:213–216

17. Huber-Spitzy VN, Czejka M, Georgiew L, et al. Penetration of norfloxacin into the aqueous humor of the human eye. Invest Ophthalmol Vis Sci 1992;33:1723–1726

18. Borrmann L, Tang-Liu DD, Kann J, et al. Ofloxacin in human serum, urine, and tear film after topical application. Cornea 1992;11:226–230

19. Leibowitz HM. Clinical evaluation of ciprofloxacin 0.3% ophthalmic solution for treatment of bacterial keratitis. Am J Ophthalmol 1991;112:34S–47S

20. Sawusch MR, O'Brien TP, Dick JD, Gottsch JD. Use of collagen corneal shields in treatment of bacterial keratitis. Am J Ophthalmol 1988;106:279–281

21. Katz HR, Cytryn AS, Parks DJ. Aqueous and vitreous levels of ciprofloxacin after subconjunctival injection in the rabbit. Invest Ophthalmol Vis Sci 1992;33:1014

22. Rootman D, Savage P, Hasany S, Basu PK. The toxicity and pharmacokinetics of intravitreal ciprofloxacin in rabbit eyes. Invest Ophthalmol Vis Sci 1991;32:1171

23. Pearson PA, Hollins J, Ashton P. Pharmacokinetics of intravitreal ciprofloxacin. Invest Ophthalmol Vis Sci 1992;33:726

24. Kaplan HJ, Cytryn AS, Parks DJ, Katz HR. Vitreous levels of ciprofloxacin after intravitreal injection in the rabbit. Invest Ophthalmol Vis Sci 1992;33:729

25. Hooper DC, Wolfson JS. The fluoroquinolones: pharmacology, clinical uses, and toxicities in humans. Antimicrob Agents Chemother 1985;28:716–721

26. Mounier M, Ploy MC, Chauvin M, et al. Etude de la penetration intraoculaire de l'ofloxacine chez l'homme et le lapin. Pathol Biol (Paris) 1992;40:529–533

27. Bron A, Talon D, Delbosc B, et al. La penetration intracamerulaire de la pefloxacine chez l'homme. J Fr Ophtalmol 1986;9:317–321

28. Salvanet A, Fisch A, Lafaix C, et al. Perfloxacin concentrations in human aqueous humour and lens. J Antimicrob Chemother 1986;18:199–201

29. Fern AI, Sweeney G, Doig M, Lindsay G. Penetration of ciprofloxacin into aqueous humour. Trans Ophthalmol Soc UK 1986;105:650

30. Luthy R, Joos B, Gassmann F. Penetration of ciprofloxacin into the human eye. In: Neu HC, Weuta H, eds. Proceedings of the first international ciprofloxacin workshop. Amsterdam: Excerpta Medica, 1985:192–196

31. Mounier M, Adenis JP, Denis P. Penetration intraoculaire de la ciprofloxacine apres perfusion et prise orale. Pathol Biol (Paris) 1988;36:724–727
32. El Baba FZ, Trousdale MD, Gauderman WJ, et al. Intravitreal penetration of oral ciprofloxacin in humans. Ophthalmology 1992;99:483–486
33. Keren G, Alhalel A, Bartov E, et al. The intravitreal penetration of orally administered ciprofloxacin in humans. Invest Ophthalmol Vis Sci 1991;32:2388–2392
34. Trucksis M, Hooper DC, Wolfson JS. Emerging resistance to fluoroquinolones in staphylococci: an alert. Ann Intern Med 1991;114:424–426
35. Piddock LJV, Wise R. The selection and frequency of streptococci with decreased susceptibility to ofloxacin compared with other quinolones. J Antimicrob Chemother 1988;22:45S–51S
36. Crumplin GC, Odell M. Development of resistance to ofloxacin. Drugs 1987;34: 1S–8S
37. Mitsui Y, Matsuda H, Miyajima T, et al. Therapeutic effects of ofloxacin eye drops (DE-055) on external infection of the eye. Multicentral double blind test. Jpn Rev Clin Ophthalmol 1986;80:1813
38. Gwon A. Ofloxacin vs tobramycin for the treatment of external ocular infection. Arch Ophthalmol (in press)
39. Bron AJ, Leber G, Rizk SNM, et al. Ofloxacin compared with chloramphenicol in the management of external ocular infection. Br J Ophthalmol 1991;75:675–679
40. Leibowitz HM. Antibacterial effectiveness of ciprofloxacin 0.3% ophthalmic solution in the treatment of bacterial conjunctivitis. Am J Ophthalmol 1991;112:29S– 33S
41. Vogel R, Laibowitz R, Castan R, et al. A placebo controlled trial of norfloxacin ophthalmic solution (NFX) in acute bacterial conjunctivitis (ABC). Invest Ophthalmol Vis Sci 1992;33:937
42. Tonjum AM. Effects of benzalkonium chloride upon the corneal epithelium studied with scanning electron microscopy. Acta Ophthalmol (Copenh) 1975;53:358–366
43. Rucker I, Kettrey R, Bach F, Zeleznick L. A safety test for contact lens wetting solutions: evaluation of currently available solutions. Ann Ophthalmol 1972;4: 1000
44. Adams J, Wilcox MJ, Trousdale MD, et al. Morphologic and physiologic effects of artificial tear formulations on corneal epithelial derived cells. Cornea 1992;11: 234–241
45. Cutarelli PE, Lass JH, Lazarus HM, et al. Topical fluoroquinolones: antimicrobial activity and in vivo corneal epithelial toxicity. Curr Eye Res 1991;10:557–563
46. Stevens SX, Fouraker BD, Jensen HG. Intraocular safety of ciprofloxacin. Arch Ophthalmol 1991;109:1737–1743
47. Gootz TD, Barrett JF, Sutcliffe JA. Inhibitory effects of quinolone antibacterial agents on eucaryotic topoisomerases and related test systems. Antimicrob Agents Chemother 1990;34:8–12
48. Halkin H. Adverse effects of the fluoroquinolones. Rev Infect Dis 1988;10:258S
49. Limberg MB. A review of bacterial keratitis and bacterial conjunctivitis. Am J Ophthalmol 1991;112:2S–9S
50. Jones DB. A plan for antimicrobial therapy in bacterial keratitis. Trans Am Acad Ophthalmol Otolaryngol 1975;79:95
51. Arffa RC. Grayson's diseases of the cornea, ed 3. St Louis: Mosby, 1991:163–198
52. Charlton JF, Kniska A, Chao GM, et al. Stability of topical fortified antibiotic solutions. Invest Ophthalmol Vis Sci 1992;33:937
53. Kaufman AH, Darrell RW, Shieh E, et al. Treatment of methicillin-resistant *Staphylococcus aureus* keratitis in rabbits with ciprofloxacin, norfloxacin, ofloxacin, vancomycin and cefazolin. Invest Ophthalmol Vis Sci 1991;32:1171
54. Roussel TJ, Osato MS, Robinson MN, et al. Resistant *Pseudomonas* keratitis. J Ocul Ther Surg 1984;3:136–138

55. Gelender H, Rettich C. Gentamicin-resistant *Pseudomonas aeruginosa* corneal ulcers. Cornea 1984;3:21–26

56. Darrell RW, Modak S, Fox CL. Norfloxacin and silver norfloxacin in the treatment of *Pseudomonas* corneal ulcer in the rabbit. Trans Am Ophthalmol Soc 1984;82: 75–87

57. Darrell RW, Menon A, Modak S, Fox CL. Topical norfloxacin in the treatment of *Staphylococcus aureus* corneal ulcer in the rabbit. Cornea 1986;5:205–209

58. Callegan MC, Hobden JA, Hill JM, et al. Chemotherapy of methicillin-sensitive and methicillin-resistant *Staphylococcus aureus* keratitis in the rabbit. Invest Ophthalmol Vis Sci 1992;33:935

59. Meredith TA. Prevention of postoperative infection. Arch Ophthalmol 1991;109: 944–945

60. Speaker MG, Milch FA, Shak MK, et al. Role of external bacterial flora in the pathogenesis of acute postoperative endophthalmitis. Ophthalmology 1991;98: 639–650

61. Forster AK, Abbott RL, Gelender H. Management of infectious endophthalmitis. Ophthalmology 1980;87:313–319

62. Tamura O, Abe M, Inoue S, Inoue S. Preoperative sterilization and prevention of postoperative infection by ofloxacin. Jpn Rev Clin Ophthalmol 1986;80:1104–1116

63. Campochiaro PA, Conway BP. Aminoglycoside toxicity—a survey of retinal specialists: implications for ocular use. Arch Ophthalmol 1991;109:946–950

64. Bron A. Apport des quinolones en ophtalmologie. In: Adenis JP, Denis F, Bron A, et al, eds. Infections et inflammations du segment anterieur de l'oeil. Paris: Merck Sharp & Dohme-Chibret, 1989:115–129

65. Salvanet-Bouccara A, Dubayle P, Forestier F, et al. Vers une strategie raisonnee du traitement des endophtalmies bacteriennes post-operatoires. J Fr Ophtalmol 1986;9:523–532

New Horizons in Antibacterial Antibiotics

Dan B. Jones, M.D.

The constant search for new antimicrobial agents is necessitated by the evolving limitations of current therapy in the management of serious infections. New antimicrobial agents must be developed to deal effectively with the appearance of new pathogens, the emergence of resistant organisms, the new pathogenic roles of familiar organisms, and the evolution of unique infections among immunosuppressed individuals, particularly those infected with the human immunodeficiency virus. Delayed recognition of toxicity of established compounds and adverse interactions among other new chemotherapeutic agents are additional factors.

The opportunity to use newly discovered antibiotics for ocular infections evolves by one of several mechanisms: (1) introduction of the agent as an ophthalmic formulation (e.g., ciprofloxacin eye drops for bacterial conjunctivitis and keratitis); (2) development of a systemic agent primarily for an ocular infection (e.g., intravenous foscarnet for cytomegaloviral retinitis); (3) utilization of the standard formulation and dosage of an agent for ocular infections caused by the same organism or class of organisms for which the antibiotic was developed (e.g., oral azithromycin for chlamydial conjunctivitis); or (4) modification of the standard formulation for an ophthalmic preparation (e.g., fluconazole eye drops for fungal keratitis).

Antibacterial agents comprise at least 18 classes (Table 1). The principal classes in which new developments have potentially important applications for use in ocular infections are the cephalosporins, beta-lactamase inhibitors, macrolides, glycopeptides, and fluoroquinolones. The new fluoroquinolone antibiotics are the subject of the chapter, "Role of the Fluoroquinolones in Ophthalmology." Notably, few advancements have emerged among other classes of antibacterial agents that have previously provided important antibiotics for ocular infections, namely the penicillins and aminoglycosides.

Table 1 *Classes of Antibacterial Agents*

Penicillins	Tetracyclines
Cephalosporins	Chloramphenicol
Beta-lactamase inhibitors	Lincosamides
	Aminoglycosides
Carbapenems	Aminocyclitols
Monobactams	Metronidazole
Macrolides	Sulfonamides
Glycopeptides	Trimethoprim
Rifamycins	Fluoroquinolones
Peptolide	

■ Cephalosporins

Cephalosporins are broad-spectrum beta-lactam antibiotics that have the same mechanism of action as penicillin to inhibit synthesis of the cell wall of susceptible organisms through interference with the peptidoglycan cross-linkage. Variability of the spectrum of activity, susceptibility to beta-lactamases, protein binding, pharmacokinetic properties, and toxicity of the cephalosporins is achieved by substitutions on the beta-lactam and dihydrothiazine rings of the basic nucleus of the molecule. Cephalosporins are traditionally considered in three groups (referred to as *generations*) based on their spectrum of activity. Cefazolin, a first-generation cephalosporin, has been used in ocular infections primarily as an alternate intravenous antibiotic for staphylococcal and streptococcal infections in individuals allergic to penicillin and as the preferred initial topical antibiotic in bacterial keratitis, either alone or in combination with gentamicin or tobramycin. The emergence of methicillin-resistant strains of staphylococci recently led to the substitution of vancomycin for cefazolin for intravitreal therapy in exogenous bacterial endophthalmitis and prompted others to consider vancomycin as the preferred initial topical agent in bacterial keratitis.

Third-generation cephalosporins offer distinct advantages over cefazolin in the initial therapy of severe bacterial keratitis in which organisms are not detected in corneal smears or in which gram-negative bacilli are suspected. Strains of *Pseudomonas aeruginosa* and other gram-negative bacilli may be more susceptible to third-generation cephalosporins than to aminoglycosides, such as gentamicin and tobramycin. The combination of a third-generation cephalosporin and an aminoglycoside may provide additive or synergistic antimicrobial effect against *P. aeruginosa* and other gram-negative bacilli and prevent emergence of resistance.

Ceftazidime is a third-generation cephalosporin with potent activity against gram-negative bacilli, including *P. aeruginosa,* and *Serratia, Enterobacter,* and *Proteus* species, and moderate activity against anaerobes. It has a low degree of protein binding (17%) and a high level of penetration into cerebrospinal fluid (mean, 9.8 µg/ml) after intravenous administration [1]. In a rabbit model of keratitis, topical ceftazidime (50 mg/ml) was equally effective as cefazolin (50 mg/ml) in the treatment of *Staphylococcus aureus* and *Streptococcus pneumoniae* keratitis and as effective as tobramycin (14 mg/ml) in *P. aeruginosa* keratitis [2]. Ceftazidime was also effective but less active than vancomycin (50 mg/ml) in methicillin-resistant *S. aureus* keratitis. Topical ceftazidime (50 mg/ml) has been used successfully at the Cullen Eye Institute in selected cases of human keratitis caused by *S. pneumoniae, P. aeruginosa, Hemophilus influenzae,* and *Alcaligenes* species.

Ceftazidime should be considered an alternate topical antibiotic in the initial management of suspected bacterial keratitis, either alone or in combination with gentamicin or tobramycin. Use of ceftazidime alone avoids the risk of corneal and conjunctival toxicity associated with topical aminoglycosides [3]. Others have recommended ceftazidime as the single intraocular agent in bacterial endophthalmitis based on its spectrum of activity and the avoidance of risk of macular infarction associated with gentamicin toxicity [4]. Of note, ceftazidime has been recommended as single-drug therapy or in combination with an aminoglycoside with or without vancomycin for initial empirical treatment of febrile neutropenic patients. A recent randomized prospective study [5] and meta-analysis of published studies [6] suggested that ceftazidime is appropriate initial monotherapy for febrile neutropenic patients.

■ Beta-Lactamase Inhibitors

Beta-lactamase inhibitors have a high, irreversible affinity for bacterial beta-lactamases and thereby prevent their hydrolytic activity on penicillins and cephalosporins. The concept of combining a beta-lactamase inhibitor with penicillins and cephalosporins originated to increase the activity of the antibiotic against resistant bacteria that produce beta-lactamases while retaining the spectrum of activity and unique pharmacokinetic properties of the penicillin or cephalosporin. Table 2 lists the currently available and investigational combinations of beta-lactamase antibiotics and beta-lactamase inhibitors.

The combination of ticarcillin and clavulanic acid was released for clinical use as a parenteral agent in 1985, yet has received little attention for use in ocular infections. Ticarcillin is an extended-spectrum carboxypenicillin that is active against a variety of gram-negative bacilli, including *P. aeruginosa* and *Enterobacter* and *Proteus* species. Ticarcillin possesses the same antibacterial activity against staphylococci and streptococci as does ampicillin. The addition of clavulanic acid to ticarcillin increases its antibiotic activity against beta-lactamase-producing strains of *S. aureus, Neisseria gonorrhoeae, H. influenzae, Bacteroides* species, and others. Methicillin-

Table 2 *Beta-lactam Antibiotics Combined with Beta-lactamase Inhibitors*

		Formulation	
Agents	Trade name	Oral	Parenteral
Amoxicillin–clavulanic acid	Amoxil, others	+	
Ampicillin-sulbactam	Unasyn		+
Ticarcillin–clavulanic acid	Timentin		+
Piperacillin-tazobactam	—		+
Cefoperazone-sulbactam	—		+

resistant staphylococci are also resistant to ticarcillin–clavulanic acid. For empirical initial therapy of severe bacterial infection of the cornea, soft tissues of the eyelids, or orbit, ticarcillin–clavulanic acid is a rational alternative to cefazolin in combination with an aminoglycoside or third-generation cephalosporin. Ticarcillin may be effective against aminoglycoside-resistant strains of *P. aeruginosa* and may provide additive effect with tobramycin or gentamicin against susceptible strains of *P. aeruginosa*.

The addition of sulbactam to ampicillin increased the activity of ampicillin against beta-lactamase-producing strains of *S. aureus, H. influenzae, Neisseria* species, and others. As ampicillin penetrates well into extracellular fluids and tissues, ampicillin-sulbactam is a rational alternative intravenous antibiotic for preseptal cellulitis, orbital cellulitis associated with paranasal sinusitis, and dacryocystitis likely caused by gram-positive cocci with a probability of beta-lactamase strains, particularly *H. influenzae*.

■ Macrolides

Erythromycin is a standard, widely used macrolide antibiotic because of its relative lack of toxicity and good activity against staphylococci, streptococci, *H. influenzae, Legionella pneumophila, Chlamydia trachomatis, Mycoplasma pneumoniae*, and *Campylobacter jejuni*. Oral erythromycin is the preferred alternate agent for the treatment of chlamydial conjunctivitis in individuals in whom a tetracycline is not indicated, such as women in the last half of pregnancy, nursing mothers, newborns, and children to age 8 years. Erythromycin ophthalmic ointment is commonly used to treat chronic staphylococcal blepharitis and mild bacterial conjunctivitis.

Macrolide antibiotics contain a lactose ring to which are attached one or more deoxy sugars. Macrolide antibiotics inhibit protein synthesis by binding to the 50S subunit of bacterial ribosomes, thereby increasing the dissociation of peptidyl-tRNA from the ribosomes. A unique property of macrolide antibiotics is the ability to penetrate polymorphonuclear leukocytes, macrophages, and lymphocytes, which has important implications in the treatment of infections caused by *Chlamydia, Mycobacterium, Toxoplasma,* and other organisms [7]. Modification of the size and substitution pattern of the lactose ring has led to the development of important new macrolide antibiotics with potential for use in ocular infections.

Clarithromycin

Clarithromycin is a 6-methoxy derivative of erythromycin that is two to four or more times more active than erythromycin against *C. trachomatis* and susceptible staphylococci and streptococci [8]. Clarithromycin is also more active than erythromycin against *Borrelia burgdorferi,* the causative agent of Lyme disease [8]. The single modification in the lactose ring renders clarithromycin more resistant than erythromycin to acid degradation in the stomach, thereby reducing gastrointestinal toxicity and improving the bioavailability of the drug. Clarithromycin is well absorbed from the gastrointestinal tract, achieves peak blood levels in 2 hours, and has a serum half-life of 5 to 7 hours [9]. It is currently available as 250-mg and 500-mg tablets (Biaxin) and approved for treatment of respiratory, skin, and soft-tissue infections.

Clarithromycin may be an effective topical or systemic agent in the treatment of ocular infections caused by nontuberculous mycobacteria, particularly *M. chelonae* and *M. fortuitum* keratitis. Clarithromycin was 10 to 50 times more active in vitro than erythromycin and 4 to 8 times more active than other new macrolide antibiotics, azithromycin and roxithromycin, against 55 strains of *M. chelonae* [9]. The minimum inhibitory concentration of clarithromycin for 90% of strains tested was 0.25 μg/ml for isolates of *M. chelonae* subspecies *chelonae* and 0.5 μg/ml for subspecies *abscessus*. Similarly, clarithromycin, azithromycin, and roxithromycin were more active than erythromycin against the majority of tested strains of *M. fortuitum*. Clarithromycin may also be effective in the treatment of *M. avium* complex infections in patients with the acquired immunodeficiency syndrome (AIDS) [9–12].

Azithromycin

Azithromycin differs from erythromycin by substitution of a tertiary nitrogen group at position 9a of the 15-membered lactose ring. This modification provides a prolonged serum half-life (41 hours), superior tissue distribution with high peak levels, and extended mean residence time [7, 13]. After a single 500-mg dose, concentrations in tissue are 400 times that achieved in serum [14]. Because of its remarkable pharmacokinetic properties, azithromycin can be administered as a single daily dose. Although azithromycin possesses better stability than erythromycin in the presence of acidic pH, each dose should be taken at least 1 hour before or 2 hours after a meal.

Azithromycin is less active than erythromycin against staphylococci and streptococci, but it is more active against *H. influenzae, L. pneumophila,* and *B. burgdorferi.* It also is comparable to erythromycin and tetracycline against *C. trachomatis* and *C. pneumoniae* [15]. A single 1-gm dose of azithromycin was as effective as a 7-day course of doxycycline for uncomplicated chlamydial genital infection [16].

Azithromycin is available as 250-mg capsules (Zithromax) and has been approved for treatment of respiratory, skin, and soft-tissue infections and chlamydial urethritis and cervicitis. The recommended dosage for chlamydial genital infections is 1 gm once. A clinical trial is currently being conducted to compare the efficacy of a single 1-gm dose of azithromycin to doxycycline, 100 mg twice daily for 7 days, in chlamydial conjunctivitis. If effective, the prolonged half-life, high levels in tissue, and single-dose regimen are distinct advantages for azithromycin, particularly in terms of greater patient compliance. In addition, azithromycin may provide adequate treatment for concurrent *N. gonorrhoeae* and *M. pneumoniae* genital infections. Recent in vitro and animal studies suggest that azithromycin may also be effective in toxoplasma infections [8]. Other novel macrolide antibiotics, such as roxithromycin, flurithromycin, dirithromycin, and rokitamycin, may prove to have unique properties of benefit for use in ocular infections.

■ Glycopeptides

Vancomycin is a complex glycopeptide antibiotic that has assumed major therapeutic importance due to the frequency of infections caused by beta-lactam-resistant gram-positive organisms, particularly methicillin-resistant staphylococci. Vancomycin inhibits the biosynthesis of peptidoglycan, the major structural polymer of the bacterial cell wall; alters the permeability of the cytoplasmic membrane; and may impair RNA synthesis [17]. Resistance to vancomycin is rare [17, 18].

In systemic and soft-tissue infections, vancomycin is the drug of choice for treatment of methicillin-resistant staphylococci and is the preferred alternate agent in serious staphylococcal and streptococcal infections in individuals intolerant of beta-lactam antibiotics. Vancomycin is the preferred antibiotic for intravitreal injection for treatment of endophthalmitis caused by gram-positive cocci and, in combination with an aminoglycoside, enhances the activity against *Enterococcus faecalis* and *Bacillus cereus* [19]. Vancomycin is also widely recommended for topical treatment of bacterial keratitis caused by gram-positive cocci, for systemic treatment of endophthalmitis and soft-tissue infections caused by gram-positive cocci and, in combination with gentamicin, for prophylaxis in tissue culture media for corneal storage. A disadvantage for use of topical or subconjunctival vancomycin is the toxicity associated with the low-pH and low-osmolarity solutions prepared with sterile water for injection [20]. Use of saline or a phosphate-buffered artificial tear preparation improves patient tolerance of topical vancomycin (50 mg/ml).

Teicoplanin is a new glycopeptide antibiotic that is similar to vancomycin in structure, mode of action, and spectrum of activity [21, 22]. Teicoplanin, however, is highly protein-bound (>90%), has a longer half-life in serum (>50 hours), may be given intramuscularly as well as intravenously, and may have less vestibular toxicity and ototoxicity [22]. Teicoplanin is effective as once-daily intravenous therapy for deep-seated bone and joint infections caused by *S. aureus,* coagulase-negative staphylococci, and streptococci [22]; catheter-associated infections caused by gram-positive cocci in patients with various hematological disorders [23]; and in various other soft-tissue, urinary tract, and upper respiratory infections [24]. Teicoplanin has excellent potential as a safe and effective agent against ocular infections caused by gram-positive cocci, and the properties of the compound may simplify its preparation and administration for corneal and intraocular infection.

■ Conclusion

Multiple challenges await new antibiotic development. Innate and acquired antimicrobial resistance will increase among common and new ocular pathogens. New plasmid-mediated enzymes will confer resistance to novel beta-lactam and other antibiotics. Complex adverse reactions will emerge, no doubt enhanced by interactions among antimicrobial and other chemotherapeutic agents. In addition to discovering new antimicrobial compounds, we must develop effective methods of targeted drug delivery, systems to eradicate biofilms, and applications of biological therapy and immunotherapy to prevent and treat ocular infectious diseases successfully.

This work was supported in part by the Sid W. Richardson Foundation, Fort Worth, TX, and Research to Prevent Blindness, New York, NY.

■ References

1. Gustaferro CA, Steckelbert JM. Cephalosporin antimicrobial agents and related compounds. Mayo Clin Proc 1991;66:1064–1073
2. Mills RA, Osato MS, Pyron M, Jones DB. Efficacy of topical ceftazidime in experimental bacterial keratitis. Invest Ophthalmol Vis Sci 1992;33:935
3. Davison CR, Tuft SJ, Dark JKG. Conjunctival necrosis after administration of topical fortified aminoglycosides. Am J Ophthalmol 1991;111:690–693
4. Campochiaro PA, Green WR. Toxicity of intravitreous ceftazidime in primate retina. Invest Ophthalmol Vis Sci 1992;33:726

5. Sanders JW, Powe NR, Moore RD. Ceftazidime monotherapy for empiric treatment of febrile neutropenic patients: a metaanalysis. J Infect Dis 1991;164:907–916

6. Ramphal R, Bolger M, Oblon DJ, et al. Vancomycin is not an essential component of the initial empiric treatment regimen for febrile neutropenic patients receiving ceftazidime: a randomized prospective study. Antimicrob Agents Chemother 1992; 36:1062–1067

7. Kirst HA, Sides GD. New directions for macrolide antibiotics: pharmacokinetics and clinical efficacy. Antimicrob Agents Chemother 1989;33:1419–1422

8. Kirst HA, Sides GD. New directions for macrolide antibiotics: structural modifications and in vitro studies. Antimicrob Agents Chemother 1989;33:1413–1418

9. Brown BA, Wallace RJ, Onyi GO, et al. Activities of four macrolides, including clarithromycin, against *Mycobacterium fortuitum, Mycobacterium chelonae,* and *M. chelonae*-like organisms. Antimicrob Agents Chemother 1992;36:180–184

10. Dautzenberg BC, Truffot C, Legris S, et al. Activity of clarithromycin against *Mycobacterium avium* infection in patients with acquired immune deficiency syndrome. Am Rev Respir Dis 1991;144:564–569

11. Young LS, Wiviott L, Wu M, et al. Azithromycin reduces *Mycobacterium avium* complex (MAC) bacteremia and relieves its symptoms in patients with AIDS [abstr 294]. Program Abstracts from the Thirty-First Interscience Conference on Antimicrobial Agents, 1991

12. De Lalla F, Maserati R, Scarpellini P, et al. Clarithromycin-ciprofloxacin-amikacin for therapy of *Mycobacterium avium-Mycobacterium intracellulare* bacteremia in patients with AIDS. Antimicrob Agents Chemother 1992;36:1567–1569

13. Azoulay-Dupuis E, Vallee E, Bedos Jean-Pierre, et al. Prophylactic therapeutic activities of azithromycin in a mouse model of pneumococcal pneumonia. Antimicrob Agents Chemother 1991;35:1024–1028

14. Walsh M, Kappas EW, Quinn TC. In vitro evaluation of CP-62, 993, erythromycin, clindamycin, and tetracycline against *Chlamydia trachomatis.* Antimicrob Agents Chemother 1987;31:811–812

15. Welsh LE, Gaydos CA, Quinn TA. In vitro evaluation of activities of azithromycin, erythromycin, and tetracycline against *Chlamydia trachomatis* and *Chlamydia pneumoniae.* Antimicrob Agents Chemother 1992;36:291–294

16. Stamm WE. Azithromycin in the treatment of uncomplicated genital chlamydial infections. Am J Med 1991;(suppl 3A):19S–22S

17. Wilhelm MP. Vancomycin. Mayo Clin Proc 1991;66:1165–1170

18. Schwalbe RS, Stapleton JT, Gilligan PH. Emergence of vancomycin resistance in coagulase-negative staphylococci. N Engl J Med 1987;316:927–931

19. Pflugfelder SC, Hernandez E, Fliesler SJ, et al. Intravitreal vancomycin. Arch Ophthalmol 1987;105:831–837

20. Fleischer AB, Hoover DL, Khan JA, et al. Topical vancomycin formulation for methicillin-resistant *Staphylococcus epidermidis* blepharoconjunctivitis. Am J Ophthalmol 1986;101:283–287

21. Peetermans WE, Hoogeterp JJ, Hazekamp-van Dokkum AM, et al. Antistaphylococcal activities of teicoplanin and vancomycin in vitro and in an experimental infection. Antimicrob Agents Chemother 1990;34:1869–1874

22. Greenberg RN. Treatment of bone, joint and vascular-access-associated gram-positive bacterial infections with teicoplanin. Antimicrob Agents Chemother 1990; 34:2392–2397

23. Smith SR, Cheesbrough J, Spearing R, Davies JM. Randomized prospective study comparing vancomycin with teicoplanin in the treatment of infections associated with Hickman catheters. Antimicrob Agents Chemother 1989;33:1193–1197

24. Stille W, Sietzen W, Dieterich HA, Fell JJ. Clinical efficacy and safety of teicoplanin. J Antimicrob Chemother 1988;21(suppl A):69–79

Index

U.S. Postal Service Statement of Ownership, Management and Circulation (required by 39 U.S.C. 3685). 1A. Title of publication: INTERNATIONAL OPHTHALMOLOGY CLINICS. 1B. Publication no.: 00208167. 2. Date of filing: October 1, 1992. 3. Frequency of issue: quarterly. 3A. No. of issues published annually: 4. 3B. Annual subscription price: $86.00. 4. Complete mailing address of known office of publication (street, city, county, state and ZIP code) (not printers): 34 Beacon Street, Boston, Suffolk County, Massachusetts 02108-1493. 5. Complete mailing address of the headquarters or general business offices of the publishers (not printers): 34 Beacon Street, Boston, Suffolk County, Massachusetts 02108-1493. 6. Full names and complete mailing address of publisher, editor, and managing editor (this item *must not* be blank): Publisher (name and complete mailing address): Little, Brown and Company, Inc., 34 Beacon Street, Boston, Massachusetts 02108-1493. Editor (name and complete mailing address): Gilbert Smolin, MD, and Mitchell Friedlaender, MD, 1001 Sneath Lane, Room 206, San Bruno, CA 94066. Managing Editor (name and complete mailing address): Sherri Frank, Little, Brown and Company, 34 Beacon Street, Boston, Massachusetts 02108-1493. 7. Owner (If owned by a corporation, its name and address must be stated and also immediately thereunder the names and addresses of stockholders owning or holding 1 percent or more of total amount of stock. If not owned by a corporation, the names and addresses of the individual owners must be given. If owned by a partnership or other unincorporated firm, its name and address, as well as that of each individual must be given. If the publication is published by a nonprofit organization, its name and address must be stated.) (Item must be completed): Full name: Little, Brown and Company (Incorporated). Complete mailing address: 34 Beacon Street, Boston, Massachusetts 02108-1493; The Time Inc. Book Company, Rockefeller Center, New York, New York 10020, which is a wholly owned subsidiary of Time Warner Inc., Rockefeller Center, New York, NY 10020. To the best of Time Warner's knowledge, the names and addresses of stockholders owning or holding one percent or more of the stock of Time Warner Inc. are as follows: Time Warner Inc., Common Stock (as of 6/2/92 unless otherwise indicated); *The Capital Group, Inc., 333 South Hope Street, Los Angeles, CA 90071 (as of December 31, 1991); *The Depository Trust Company, P.O. Box 20, Bowling Green Station, New York, NY 10274; The Henry Luce Foundation, Inc., 111 West 50th Street, New York, NY 10020; *The Equitable Life Assurance Society of the United States, 787 Seventh Avenue, New York, NY 10019 (as of 12/31/91). Time Warner Inc., Series C 8¾% Convertible Exchangeable Preferred Stock and/or Series D 11% Convertible Exchangeable Preferred Stock (as of 8/17/92 unless otherwise indicated): BHC Communications Inc., 600 Madison Avenue, New York, NY 10022-1615; Chris Craft Television Inc., 600 Madison Avenue, New York, NY 10022-1615; United Television Inc., 8501 Wilshire Blvd., Suite 340, Beverly Hills, CA 90211-3119; *The Depository Trust Company, P.O. Box 20, Bowling Green Station, New York, NY 10274-0020; *Fayez Sarofim & Co., 2907 Two Houston Center, Houston, TX 77010 (as of 12-31-91); *Eagle Asset Management Inc., 880 Carillon Parkway, P.O. Box 10520, St. Petersburg, FL 33733-0520 (as of 12-31-91). EBENCO, P.O. Box 2140, Pasadena, CA 91102; Steven J. Ross, 75 Rockefeller Plaza, New York, NY 10019 (*Held for the account of one or more security holders.) 8. Known bondholders, mortgagees, and other security holders owning or holding 1 percent or more of total amount of bonds, mortgages or other securities (if there are none, so state): *The Depository Trust Company, P.O. Box 20, Bowling Green Station, New York, NY 10274 (as of 9/13/91; *Held for the account of one or more security holders.) 9. For completion by nonprofit organizations authorized to mail at special rates (Section 423.12, DMM only). The purpose, function, and nonprofit status of this organization and the exempt status for Federal income tax purposes (Check one): (1) Has not changed during preceding 12 months; (2) Has changed during preceding 12 months (If changed, publisher must submit explanation of change with this statement.): None. 10. Extent and nature of circulation: A. Total no. copies (net press run): average no. copies each issue during preceding 12 months, 2911; actual no. copies of single issue published nearest to filing date, 2727. B. Paid circulation: 1. Sales through dealers and carriers, street vendors and counter sales: average no. copies each issue during preceding 12 months, 56; actual no. copies of single issue published nearest to filing date, 59. 2. Mail subscription: average no. copies each issue during preceding 12 months, 1971; actual no. copies of single issue published nearest to filing date, 1846. C. Total paid circulation (sum of 10B1 and 10B2): average no. copies each issue during preceding 12 months, 2027; actual no. copies of single issue published nearest to filing date, 1905. D. Free distribution by mail, carrier or other means, samples, complimentary, and other free copies: average no. copies each issue during preceding 12 months, 108; actual no. copies of single issue published nearest to filing date, 157. E. Total distribution (sum of C and D): average no. copies each issue during preceding 12 months, 2135; actual no. copies of single issue published nearest to filing date, 2062. F. Copies not distributed: 1. Office use, left over, unaccounted, spoiled after printing: average no. copies each issue during preceding 12 months, 776; actual no. copies of single issue published nearest to filing date, 665. 2. Return from news agents: average no. copies each issue during preceding 12 months, none; actual no. copies of single issue published nearest to filing date, none. G. Total (sum of E, F1 and 2—should equal net press run shown in A): average no. copies each issue during preceding 12 months, 2911; actual no. copies of single issue published nearest to filing date, 2727. H. I certify that the statements made by me above are correct and complete. Signature and title of editor, publisher, business manager, or owner: Christine Finn, Business Manager.